Theresa

How To Be

Healed

And

Stay Healed

By

Desmond Thomas

Unless otherwise indicated, all scripture quotations are taken from the King James Version of the Bible.

1st Printing
How To Be Healed And Stay Healed
How to walk in the fullness of God's covenant of healing and health and how to minister that grace to others also

ISBN 0-9543083-0-1
Copyright © 2002 by Desmond A. Thomas
P.M.B 365
Freetown, Sierra Leone
West Africa

Publication by MIWORD Publishing
P.M.B. 365
Freetown, Sierra Leone
West Africa

85 William Bonney Estate
Clapham Crescent
London SW4 7JS

Designed & Illustrated By:
Chosen Graphics, London
chosengraphics@lineone.net
+44 020 8591 3154;

CONTENTS

Acknowledgements

Forward

Preface

Section I-	I AM the God that healeth thee	1
	1. The Nature of God	2
	2. 5-Fold Redemption	13
Section II-	How to receive your healing	21
	1. Faith	22
	2. Confession	27
	1. Action.	32
	2. Instantaneous and Progressive Healing	35
Section 111	How to keep your healing	41
	1. Beware of unbelief	42
	2. Beware of sin	48

Section 1V-   **How to administer healing**   53

1. Go and preach   54

2. The prayer of faith   60

3. Ask the Father in Jesus' name   63

4. Prayer of Intercession   66

5. Prayer of Agreement   69

6. Laying on of hands   72

7. Anointing with oil   74

8. The Gifts of Healing   77

Section V -   **According to your faith**
                  so be it   **83**

1. The measure you measure   84

Section V1-   **Longevity of Life**   98

Section V11   **Testimonies on Healing**   118

Acknowledgement

I thank God who has taught me His word of healing which I now share with you. All praise to God for this knowledge and testimonies in this book.

I want to thank my wife Mary for the confidence she has in me and for allowing me to spend long hours at night studying and putting this book together.

Many thanks also goes to my Bishop Rev. Abu Koroma, my Pastors Rev. Abdul Momoh, Pastor Eugene Tenga and Pastor Susan Sisay for their support. My thanks also go to every member of Flaming Evangelical Ministries UK and friends from other ministries for their support to me in the making of this book.

Last but not the least I would like to thank Trevor Saxby for doing the final proofreading of this book. God bless you all and a big thanks to you all from the bottom of my heart.

Foreword

There are many books available in many Christian Bookshops that address this serious problem of sickness that has plagued the human race for ages. This book contains pertinent principle that do not only provide the genesis of this enemy of the human race but also outline the panacea needed to deal with this satanic problem called disease. God has made the necessary provision for you to overcome every sickness that tends to destroy-mankind.

In this book Pastor Desmond has outlined the provision that God has made through His word for your healing. As you imbibe the rich spiritual contents of this book with an open heart, you will discover another horizon of healing and health that will help you to surmount every challenges that stand on your path to soundhealth.

Pastor Desmond is a seasoned Bible teacher with vast experience in the ministry. He has made available to us the principles, which he has been communicating to others during his many years in the ministry. May God bless you richly as you take the journey that will enrich your life spiritually.

Bishop Frederick Abu Koronta
President and Founder
Flaming Evangelical Ministries International

Preface

Ever since I came to know the Lord Jesus as my Saviour I have developed a strong faith, which allows me to believe whatever the Scriptures have to say about the power of Jesus Christ. Because of this faith I am not bothered about trying out what the Bible says concerning me.

I came to receive Jesus as my Healer since I was taught that it is the LORD'S will to heal. As a boy, I cut my finger very badly one day and I remember asking the LORD to heal me. By that evening, the wound had dried up. I could hardly see any trace of the cut on my finger that same evening. The following day, I was testifying in school to my biology teacher about my healing. At that time she tried to disprove the power of God to heal and argued that my finger got healed naturally because the body has power to heal itself.

I knew that that particular healing took place quicker than the natural process could take, but also learnt that God heals us also through the natural capabilities of our bodies because He made the body with the ability to heal itself. If God were not healer or concerned about our health He would not make our bodies to fight against foreign antibodies and with the power to heal itself.

When I became older and entered the ministry, I began to witness more outstanding healings than wounded fingers and headaches being healed. I began to see before my very eyes God healing the deaf and dumb as I prayed for people with such disabilities. Jesus heals yesterday, today and will still continue to heal until He comes again. Whether you are a child or an adult, if you reach out in simple faith to Him to be a Healer to you or others through your prayers, He will prove Himself to be Jehovah - Rapha: The "I AM that healeth thee".

Throughout my fifteen years of healing ministry to the sick, and having looked very closely into the subject of healing, this is my simple but sincere conclusion: God is our Healer.

—— Section I ——

I Am the God That Healeth Thee

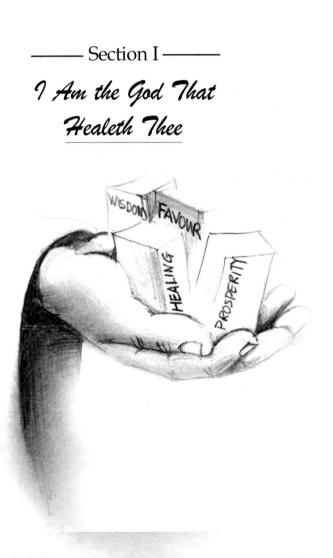

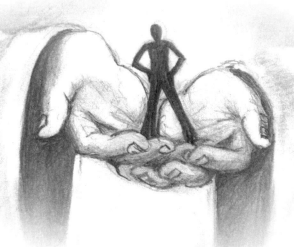

1. The Nature Of God

GOD GUARDS US
FROM SICKNESS & DISEASES

" *And said, if thou wilt diligently hearken to the voice of The LORD thy God, and wilt do that which is right in His sight, and wilt give ear to his commandments, And keep all his statutes, I will put (allow) none of These diseases upon thee, which I have brought upon the Egyptians:*

FOR I AM THE LORD THAT HEALETH THEE"

Exodus 15:26

Judging by the original Hebrew text of this scripture, the word " put " is better translated " allow " . God will not allow any sickness and disease upon the Israelites, His covenant keeping people, (which He allowed upon the Egyptians) because, it is not in accordance with His nature. He is the God who heals and not the one who afflicts people with sickness and diseases.

God made a covenant with the children of Israel to keep them from the diseases that came upon the Egyptians. These infirmities include: plagues, boils, pestilence and deaths to name a few. He also added that He was going to fulfil the number of their days with long life and health. Barrenness and miscarriages was also supposed to be absent from their midst and their children should be healthy and void of any form of deformity when He said:

" *Blessed shall be the fruit of thy body...*"
Deuteronomy 28:4

" *With long life will I satisfy him, and show him my salvation . Psalm 91:16*

" *Who forgiveth all thine iniquities; who healeth all thy diseases; Who redeemeth thy life from destruction; who crowneth thee with loving kindness and tender mercies;*

Who satisfieth thy mouth with good things; so that thy youth is renewed like the eagle's. "
Psalm 103:3-5

" *And he will love thee, and bless thee, and multiply thee: He will also bless the fruit of thy womb...*

Thou shalt be blessed above all people: there shall not be male or female barren among you, or among your cattle. And the LORD will take away from thee all sickness,

And will put none of the evil diseases of Egypt, which thou knowest, upon thee..."

Deuteronomy 7:13-15

Breaking God's covenant makes us vulnerable to sickness. As long as Israel keeps covenant with God, He was going to keep every kind of diseases from them. Note that God called them "evil diseases" , so they could not have come from God. God cannot be tempted to do evil James would let us know because evil is not in accordance with the nature of God, for God is a good God.

Though God keeps people from harm he is only covenant bound to keep His own from sickness and disease. If we are ignorant of God's covenant, the Devil can take advantage of us. If we break God's covenant we can aslo make ourselves vulnerable to the Devil.

" Let no man say when he is tempted, I am tempted of God: for God cannot be tempted with evil, neither tempteth he any man:"
James 1:13

If by any chance the Children of Israel were to transgress the commandments of God and become say idolatrous, He would keep Himself from protecting them, and would allow their enemies to afflict them. He would also not protect them from sickness and disease. Instead of them receiving a blessing to which they were called, they would become a cursed people (void of God's protection).

" The LORD shall make pestilence cleave unto thee...

The LORD shall smite thee with consumption, and with a fever,

And with an inflammation, and with extreme burning...

The LORD shall smite thee with madness, and blindness,

And astonishment of heart: (Heart attack)"

Deuteronomy 28:21,22,28

If you continue reading Deuteronomy chapter 28 you will see all the things God would allow them to suffer if they neglect His commandments. However if they repent of their sins He would forgive them, restore His covenant with them and continue to be their healer.

God Is Our Chief Doctor

God prescribed certain ceremonial preservations and rituals from 'uncleanness' and other ceremonial cleansing for the Israelites because He is their Healer. Certain practices, behavioural patterns and foods were considered unclean to keep them from being contaminated by them.

Today, a doctor can warn his patients to keep away from certain food or habits that will deter their health or cause an allergy because in his occupation he has sworn to save life. God was Israel's physician so he gave them dietary rules. His laws preserved them from sickness and diseases. The Hebrew word for 'healing' is Raphah. In fact God called Himself Jehovah - Rapha that closely associates His name to His nature.

The word Raphah actually means 'to mend by stitching, cure, heal, physician, repair thoroughly, make whole, to slacken, abate, cease'. With these words we can draw the conclusion that God is our Physician, Surgeon and healer.

We see God healing the children of Israel throughout the Old Testament. In the New Testament, God also revealed His nature in Jesus Christ whom He anointed with the Holy Spirit and power. Jesus went about doing " good " and healing all those who were oppressed by the devil. For God was with Him. *(Acts 10:38)*

I WILL

Jesus testified to the fact that He is one with the Father by saying, " I and the Father are one" . He also said that, " Whosoever hath seen me, hath seen the father also". Jesus said this for us to know that He is the very image and likeness of the Father identifying Himself with the Father in the healing business.

" *Surely he hath borne our griefs and carried our sorrows:*" *Isaiah 53:4*

The will of Jesus is the will of the Father because He came to do God's will. That will is to heal our diseases and to carry all our sicknesses away. We are going to look at several accounts in the New Testament where Jesus Christ demonstrated His Father's healing Will.

The Man with Leprosy

" ...Lord if thou wilt, thou canst make me clean.

And Jesus put forth his hand, and touched him,

Saying, I WILL, be thou clean. And

Immediately his leprosy was cleansed "

Matthew 8:2-3

Note that Jesus said to the man " I will " . He was so willing to heal the man that His heart moved His hand towards the man and touched him. Jesus wants to give you a healing touch. Invite Him in; He wants to heal you. This man's sickness in his days was untouchable. Jesus broke the tradition of the day to meet him at the point of his need. Jesus can do the same for you.

It doesn't matter how people have detested you because of your infirmity Jesus wants to take you out of your situation if you would let Him. He said to the man with leprosy, " *I will, be thou clean"* and he was cleansed of his leprosy.

The Centurion's Servant

A Roman Centurion came to Jesus requesting him to heal his servant who was at home sick. Immediately this Roman came over to Jesus to put forth his request concerning his servant, Jesus said to him:

" *I WILL come and heal him* " *Matthew 8:7*

Jesus is the willing healer. His will is to heal everyone regardless of your past, religion, colour or status. He was even willing to go to this man's house to pray for his servant even though the man was not asking him to do that. The man just wants Jesus to speak the word only for his servant to be healed. He knew that wherever his servant is, he would be healed by the words of Jesus. Jesus said, " I will come and heal him ". Distance could not be of any hindrance either to Him or to His words because He can heal even at a distance.

Many Healed

" *When the even was come, they brought unto him many that were possessed with devils: and he cast out the spirit with his word, and HEALED ALL that were sick:*

That it might be fulfilled which was spoken by Esaias the prophet, saying, Himself took our infirmities, and bare our sicknesses "

Matthew 8:16-17

The leper was not sure whether it was the will of Jesus to heal him. He did not deny that Jesus was able to heal, but he was in doubt whether Jesus would heal HIM. He was not sure whether healing was HIS portion. However, he knew that if Jesus was willing to heal him, then he was sure to get healed. So why not try it out he must have imagined. He came to Jesus and said Jesus, "I know if you are willing you can heal me."

Jesus assured him that healing was also made available to him and that healing is his portion, and He healed him. I don't care whatever your reasons might be for not thinking that Jesus would heal you. It does not matter what sin you may have committed. The reason this man was sick might have been because of his sins - but Jesus healed him anyway. He can do the same for you if you would believe that healing belongs to you.

Jesus took all your grief and carried all your sorrows through His death on the cross for you.

" *...Is any sick among you? Let him call for the elders of the Church ... And the prayer of faith shall save the sick; and the Lord shall raise him up; and if he have committed sins, they shall be forgiven him"*

James 5:14-15

The centurion knew that Jesus has authority over sickness and diseases. As a Roman Officer, he understood authority through the power of the spoken word, so he asked Jesus to speak the word or (give the command for obedience) against his servant's sickness. He believed the sickness would obey Jesus' command because Jesus has power and dominion over sickness and diseases. This man also recognised the fact that distance does not make any difference to the spoken word of Jesus.

Space cannot prevent the authority of the word of God to take place because God fills the universe. That is why the man was not troubled about whether or not Jesus would go into his house. As far as he was concerned that would only be a waste of Jesus time: He can do it at a distance! He need not be on the spot at all. Jesus can heal you where you are. He has already spoken the words for your healing.

All you need to do is find those words in the Bible and receive them by faith. They still have the same power and Jesus is at the right hand of authority in Heaven waiting for you to declare His word for your health for Him to bring it to pass in you life. *(Hebrews 3:1)*

Jesus can heal you in your bed or your armchair. He is right there where you are sitting or lying. Your Pastor need not come to your bedside. He can pray for you over the phone and something will begin to happen to you where you are because it is the omnipresent Jehovah Rapha who heals you. The centurion just went his way and believed it was done

" ...And his servant was healed in the selfsame hour."

Matthew 8:13

The word of God makes it absolutely clear that God does heal and He would heal you. There is no two ways about it. Receive your healing now in Jesus' name.

Jairus believed in the process of laying on of hands on the sick. He believed that there is healing power in Jesus' hands. He believed all Jesus had to do was to touch his daughter. The anointing flowed through the hands of Jesus, as Jairus has believed, and His daughter was raised from the dead.

> " ...*But come and lay thy hand upon her, and she shall live* "
>
> " ...*He went in, and took her by the hand, and the maid arose* "
>
> *Matthew 9:18,25*
>
> " ...*They shall lay their hands on the sick, and they shall recover*"
>
> *Mark 16:18*

The woman with the issue of blood believed that Jesus was so anointed that His garment also carried the anointing. She believed against all odds and she was healed. She came, she touched and she was healed. That's the touch of faith.

> " *So that from his body was brought unto the sick handkerchiefs and aprons, and the diseases departed from them, and the evil spirits went out from them*"
> *Acts 19:12*

It does not matter by what process you believe your healing would come. All the processes through which healing came in the Bible all worked with maximum power and maximum effectiveness. The fact remains that Jesus heals and still heals today; for with God nothing shall be impossible.

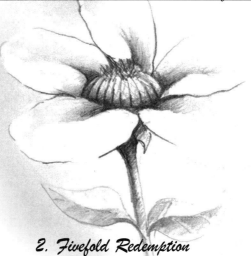

2. Fivefold Redemption

SOTERIA

The word salvation is an inclusive word. It comes from the Greek word " Soteria" which includes the aspects of deliverance, preservation and healing. Soteria does not only mean to be saved from sin, the package Jesus gave us has other things in it besides salvation from sin.

" Surely he hath borne all our griefs and carried our sorrows; yet we did esteem him stricken, smitten of God and afflicted.

But he was wounded for our transgression, he was bruised for our iniquities: the chastisement for our peace was upon him; and with his stripes we are healed "
Isaiah 53:4-5

" Christ hath redeemed us from the curse of the law, being made a curse for us: for it is written, cursed is everyone that hangeth on a tree:"   Galatians 3:13

" For ye know the grace of our Lord Jesus Christ, that, though he was rich, yet for your sakes became poor, so that ye through his poverty might be rich "
2Corinthians 8:9

From these scriptures, we can draw out five things Jesus did for us on his cross at Calvary:

1. He was wounded for our transgressions and bruised for our Iniquities - **He settled the sin problem.**

2. He bore all our griefs and carried all our sorrow and by His Stripes we are healed - **He settled the sickness problem.**

3. He was rich yet for our sakes He became poor so that through His poverty we might be rich - **He settled the poverty problem.**

4. He redeemed us from the curse of the law - **He settled the curse problem.**

5. He was chastised for our peace - **He settled the enemy problem.**

We who believe in this 5-fold redemption do know that by His stripes we were healed. *(1Peter 2:24).* We are healed people. Have you accepted Jesus Christ as your healer yet? Now is the time! Dare to receive Him as your healer, physician and surgeon?

You know tradition has taught people to think that God intends that we suffer with some kind of sickness and disease believing that it is His will for our lives. We tend to just major on salvation from sins and let whatever out there dish us with anything foul and ugly. If we can major in other areas of our salvation, as we would have with salvation from sin we would be giants on earth.

Divine Health

God healed the waters of Marah and made them sweet. *(Exodus 15:23)* Afterwards, He took Israel to Elim where there were twelve wells of water and seventy palm trees. *(Exodus 15:27)* This signifies two things. At Marah, God is our healer and at Elim, He sustains our health. In Marrah we are healed and in Elim we walk in divine health.

God does not only want to heal you, He wants you to walk in Divine health - where sickness will not touch your body. You WERE healed by the stripes of Jesus who BORE your sickness and CARRIED all your sicknesses away

According to Peter, "were healed ", "healed" and "bore" are all in past tense. Jesus had already paid the price for your healing even before the foundation of the world. It was manifested when He died over 2000 years ago on the cross of Calvary, therefore receive your healing and walk in divine health in Jesus' name.

Having eternal life is not just the ability to live forever but also the potential to live the life of the eternal God. We live like Him, have His kind of faith and if God walks in health all the time we too can walk in health all the time in Jesus' name. Amen.

One Healer and One Destroyer!

" The thief comes not, but for to steal, and to kill, and to destroy: I am come that they might have life, and that they might have it more abundantly"

John 10:10

The Devil's intentions are to kill, steal and destroy. He uses our sinful nature and habits as a means to afflict us with sickness and diseases. Viruses, bugs and also man's involvement with the earth have also brought sickness and disease upon the face of the earth but we need not fall victim of the fall. Jesus has paid the price for our healing:

" How God anointed Jesus of Nazareth with the Holy Ghost and with power: who went about doing good, and healing all that were oppressed of the devil; for God was with Him".

Acts 10:38

The Bible teaches that sicknesses and diseases are some of the oppressive acts of the devil. The devil is evil. He tries to inflict diseases on us to try to disprove the fact that God wants us to walk in health. He tries to tell us that sickness is our portion so much that when you tell people they don't need to stay sick, they think you must be very strange. Some think sickness should be an everyday thing for them.

You must at least have a sickness you can call your sickness some would imagine! My friend, you need not brand yourself with a sickness, nor do you need to be sick, because God anointed Jesus with the Holy Ghost and with power to heal all that are oppressed by the devil. This was the purpose Jesus was made manifest on this earth - to destroy the works of the Devil.

Sickness is one of such works. The whole creation is waiting for us sons of God to be made manifest in order that we might liberate it from the bondage of corruption.

" *And ought not this woman, being a daughter of Abraham, whom Satan hath bound, lo, these eighteen years, be loosed from this bond on the Sabbath day*" ? *Luke 13:16*

The above scripture let us know that Satan is the author of sickness and diseases. This woman I would say was suffering from arthritis. Here we found out that Jesus called arthritis bondage of Satan. Disease is bondage of Satan. I divide the word disease into two words because that's what exactly it is. Anything that hinders your physical well being is a dis-ease. If it causes dis-ease it is bondage of the devil; a disease.

Many sons and daughters of Abraham argue that sicknesses and diseases are God's way of punishing us. If that's the case, why do they run away from God's punishment by trying to find medical cure for it? Besides, God is a good God and I don't see how a good God can afflict or bound His own children with sickness and diseases. No earthly parent would like to do that and if we who are evil know how to give good gifts to our children I believe a good God would know better.

If you have the power to do so with your children would you do it? God knows better. God would not have come in the person of Jesus Christ destroying His own works, if sickness is an act of God. God would then become a transgressor, which He is not. *(Galatians 2:17-18)*

The Devil is the cause of all AIDS, HIV, cancers, arthritis, miscarriages, wars, genocide, earthquakes etc. God is not responsible; so don't blame it on Him. He is not responsible for the death of your loved one; Satan is responsible. You might say, isn't He running the universe? No, my friend He is not! This may baffle you, but do you know who is in charge? YOU are in charge.

The Earth was Adam's; he then sold it over to the Devil. Jesus came and took it back from the Devil and He has given the Earth back to you. If you don't do anything about yourself and your loved ones through the authority Jesus has given you in His name, nothing is going to be done about it.

" *And Jesus came and spake unto them saying, all authority is given me in Heaven and in Earth*" .

Matthew 28:18

" *Behold, I give unto you power to tread upon serpents and scorpions, and over all the power of the enemy: and nothing shall by any means hurt you*" .

Luke 10:19

" *And these signs shall follow THEM THAT BELIEVE; IN MY NAME shall they cast out devils, they shall speak with new tongues;*

They shall take up serpents; and if they drink any deadly thing, it shall not hurt them; and THEY SHALL LAY THEIR HANDS ON THE SICK, AND THEY SHALL RECOVER"

Mark 16:17-18

Jesus is talking to you, believer. He is not responsible for those that are not His. His mercies and omnipotence cover them all but He is not covenant-bound to keep them. He can only do it if we ask Him to.

" *... I am come that they might have life, and that they might have it more abundantly*" John 10:10

" *... For this purpose was the Son of God manifested, that He might destroy the works of the devil*" 1 John 3:8

" *...By his stripes ye are healed*" Isaiah 53:4

From these scriptures we find out that Jesus came to give us a life of abundance, lacking nothing. We have abundant health in Jesus. His purpose is to destroy anything that is contrary to divine health. By His stripes we were healed. Say this prayer with me just like you said the prayer of salvation when you were saved.

PRAYER

Father, I accept Jesus Christ as my healer. I believe that by His stripes I am healed. I declare that I was healed a long time ago from the time Jesus was beaten for me in Pilate's judgement hall. I was healed, I am healed and I will always be healed. Thank you for healing me Lord, I am so glad you have healed me in Jesus' name. AMEN.

Section II

How To Receive Your Healing

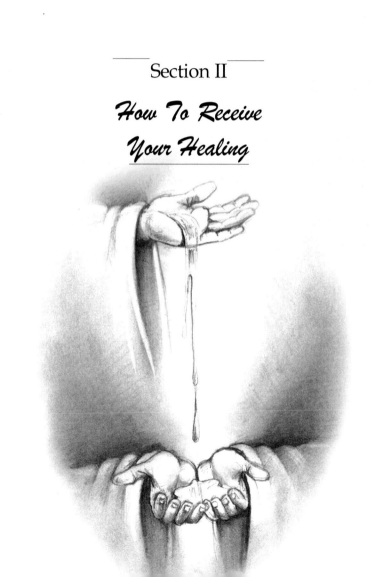

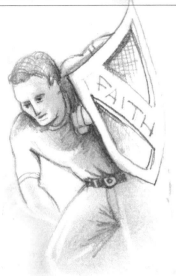

1. *Faith*

FAITH MUST HAVE ITS ANCHOR
IN THE WORD OF GOD

" And Jesus answering saith unto them, Have faith in God.

For verily I say unto you, That whosoever shall say unto this mountain, Be thou removed and be thou cast into the sea; and shall not doubt in his heart, but shall believe that those things which he saith shall come to pass; he shall have whatsoever he saith" .
Mark 11:22-23

God is our healer. Anyone who comes to God for healing MUST believe that God is healer. Faith is the first step to receiving our healing from God. If we don't believe in divine healing we would not be healed by divine means. Therefore BELIEVE IN GOD. Believing is the MUST FACTOR. In believing God, we need to understand what He has to say about our healing. Faith must have an anchor and that anchor is the word of God. Usually when you go to the hospital, the nurse or doctor will give you a leaflet to give you an understanding concerning the sickness you are faced with.

These leaflets also give you knowledge of how to treat yourself for that sickness before you can consult a doctor. The doctor then does the finishing touch when you get to his surgery.

God said that He is your healer. Look into the Word of God and see what He has to say concerning your sickness and diseases. When AIDS was first detected people did not know how it could be contracted. People invented the most absurd theories concerning AIDS until studies were carried out for people to have a perfect understanding about how it can be transmitted. People go about listening to others who have no idea about divine healing, and as a result they believe all kinds of stuff, which prevents them from receiving their healing.

Go and search the scriptures concerning these things, which are written in this book. If they are not in accordance with scriptures, don't receive them. Study all the occurrences of healings and miracles in the Bible and draw a conclusion for yourself if God is healer.

I know as you read with an open heart, your faith will develop and your healing will come because " faith comes by hearing and hearing by the word of God" . God also says, " I am the God that healeth thee." Believe that He is your Physician, Surgeon and Healer because He says so.

" But without faith it is impossible to please him; for he that cometh to God must believe that He is, and that He is a rewarder of them that diligently seek Him"

Hebrews 11:6

Faith comes by hearing God's Word

"   And a certain woman, which had an issue of blood twelve years,

And had suffered many things of many physicians, and spent all that she had, and was nothing bettered, but rather grew worse,

When she heard of Jesus"

Mark 5:25-27a

I wish the woman had heard about Jesus before she heard about all those other physicians! She could not have suffered so many things at their hand! She would not have grown worse; instead, she would have been made whole a long time ago. You could imagine all the practice that has been done in her, no wonder she grew worse. All the same, SHE HEARD OF JESUS. What could she have heard? She could have heard that He heals the sick. In fact that was what stirred up faith within her. She could have heard how Jesus lost no patient at all and how all who came to Him were healed.

What you hear will either trigger your faith or cause you to doubt. This woman heard about the healer and she was healed instantly when she met Him. Her faith caused her to reason within herself. She had lost everything she had, so she had nothing to lose now. She had to give it her best shot. She put all the faith she had into it and she was made well in an instant. Give it all the faith you have, because your healing is on the way.

This woman could have chosen to believe what other people had to say about Jesus. She could have believed that Jesus had a demon as the Pharisees believed in those days. She could have chosen to believe that Jesus was just another political freedom fighter, as some will have us believe. No, she refused to go with the wrong crowd. She chose to believe that Jesus was her healer, and she was healed.

The woman with the issue of blood believed in Jesus' clothes, the Centurion believed in His words, Jairus believed in His hands, the leper believed in His will. Wherever your faith is in Jesus, you will be made whole. Believe, for all things are possible to everyone who believes. Believe whatever the word says about Him He is nothing less than faithful to His word. He would hasten to perform His word. Aren't you glad He is not a stereotype?

2. *Confession*

CONFESSION MAKES
HEALING POSSIBLE

" That if thou shalt confess with thy mouth the Lord Jesus, and shalt believe with thy heart that God hath raised him from the dead, thou shalt be saved

For with the heart man believeth unto righteousness and with the mouth CONFESSION IS MADE UNTO SALVATION"

Romans 10 :9-10

The second step of faith for you to receive your healing is confession. Believing with your heart brings you into right standing or righteousness with God for your healing. Your believing justifies your healing, but it is your confession that brings your healing to manifestation.

The judge can declare you not guilty but if you still remain where you were once confined you make yourself a voluntary prisoner. Confession is walking your way out of that prison because the judge has declared you innocent. You must confess your faith.

God wants to hear it and Satan need to know you believe it. God has designed that confession is made unto salvation. You too need to hear your faith so that you can make your healing-way prosperous. You need to have faith in your faith.

Confession is made unto salvation. Your confession reveals your faith. Your confession precedes your action. Your confession will determine whether you are going to stay in your sickness for a long time or whether you are going to jump out of it now. Your confession determines what you are going to do next.

The Centurion's confession was:

" ... *Speak the word only, and MY SERVANT SHALL BE HEALED* "

Matthew 8:8

Jairus' confession was

" *. But come and lay thy hand upon her, AND SHE*

SHALL LIVE"
Matthew 9:18b

The leper's confession was:

" Lord if thou wilt THOU CANST MAKE ME CLEAN"

Matthew 8:2

Confess your faith and hold fast to it. Believe it and it shall come to pass. Confess that you have your healing! All these people confessed that they would be healed. They acted out their confession. You should make an actual confession of your healing before you can receive it. God's word declares that confession makes salvation possible.

You shall have whatsoever you say

" And Jesus answering saith unto them, Have faith in God.

For verily I say unto you, that whosoever shall SAY unto this mountain, Be thou removed, and be thou cast into the sea; and shall not doubt in his heart, but shall believe that THOSE THINGS WHICH HE SAITH shall come to pass; HE SHALL HAVE WHATSOEVER HE SAITH"

Mark 11:22-23

YOU SHALL HAVE WHATSOEVER YOU SAY.

Jesus didn't say: " Say what you have" . He said, " Have what you say" . Many people have willingly misunderstood this scripture. They want to believe what they want to believe, rather than believing the truth. Our confession of faith does not deny the existence of sickness in our bodies; it only denies the right of that sickness in our body, based on the finished work of Jesus Christ for our healing. Simple obedience to the principles of Gods word would result in the fulfilment of His word in our lives.

" *...For the Lord hath said, I will never leave thee, nor forsake thee. So WE MAY BOLDLY SAY, The Lord is my helper, I will not fear what man shall do unto me*"

Hebrews 13:6

Once God has spoken on your behalf (The Lord hath said, I will never leave thee, nor forsake thee) just boldly confess His words back to Him believing every report of it. Confess God's word boldly and it shall be well with you in Jesus' name.

Confess your healing. Tell it to everybody! Are you going to pray for yourself? Then tell everyone that as soon as you lay your hand on yourself you will be healed. Are you calling for the elders of your Church? Well tell everyone that as soon as the prayer of faith is said over you and as soon as you are anointed with oil, you are going to be healed.

Are you paralysed? Confess that you will walk. If you are blind, confess that you will see. Are you deaf, confess that you will hear. Are you diagnosed with cancer? Confess that it is gone, because confession is made unto salvation, and you shall have what ever you say, because Jesus " *took all your grief and carried all your sorrow*" and because, *"you shall have whatsoever you say."*

"Who his own self bare our sins in his own body on the tree, that we, being dead to sins, should live unto right-eousness: by whose stripes ye were healed"

1Peter 2:24

You are a healed person. Isn't it wonderful for you to know that you were healed? Jump out of that bed and smell the scent of fresh air. You are healed! This then leads us to the next step in completion of our healing - Action.

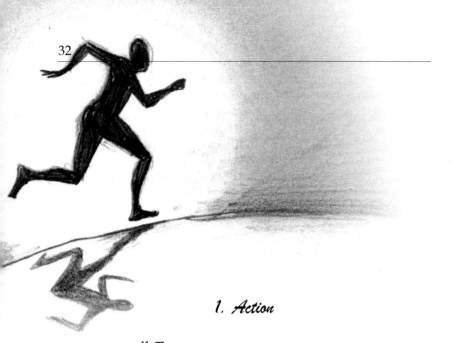

1. Action

" FAITH IS PROVED GENUINE BY CORRESPONDING ACTION "

We know that " with the heart man believes unto righteousness and with the mouth confession is made unto salvation ". For you to receive healing you must have a heart faith, mouth faith and deed faith. Faith believes with the heart, confesses with the mouth and takes the necessary action. That is what I mean by heart, mouth and action faith.

J. O. Marshall says that, " True faith is received by hearing the word of God, inspired by the anointing of the Holy Ghost, strengthened by using the word of God in prayer, released by confessing out the word and PROVED GENUINE BY CORRESPONDING ACTION"

Act out your faith. Demonstrate it. Show me your faith without your action and I will show you my faith by my actions. Your healing will come when you make the corresponding action.

The woman with the issue of blood HEARD about Jesus, she CONFESSED that if she touched Him she would be made well. She did not stop there, she had to go and touch Jesus before her healing was complete. She took the necessary faith-action. Your healing will be complete when you take the necessary ACTION.

The lame man at Lystra HEARD Paul preach and had faith to be healed after he had heard what Paul preached. Paul said, " Stand upright on your feet " and THE MAN LEAPED AND WALKED. He took the necessary ACTION and he was healed.

Ten lepers came to Jesus for healing. Jesus commanded that they go and show themselves to the priests. They were obedient to His words, AND AS THEY WERE GOING they were healed.

These people could have objected to the fact that they were healed, until they feel healed in their body. No! They did not object to their healing because their action tells me that. They believed, took the necessary action and were healed. Taking the necessary action or being obedient to the word for your healing brings about the healing you so desire.

" But be ye doers of the word and not hearers only, deceiving your own selves " .
James 1:22

Faith without action is dead being alone

It is not the hearers of the word who are justified before God but the doers of the word. If you have faith to be healed, do the things you were not able to do before. A healed man does not lie in bed when there are things to do. If you are deaf expect to hear, blind, expect to see etc. Act out your faith for faith without works (action) is dead being alone.

Your action is what demonstrates your faith. It is what proves you have faith to be healed. Your action must demonstrate the faith you have in your heart. What you believe you must confess (or say) and what you say you must act. Be a man or woman of your word and let your word be your work. You don't have to feel anything to receive anything from God. Faith is not a feeling but action, feeling may not be there, feeling is only a bonus.

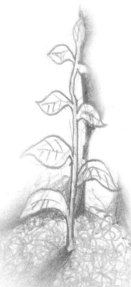

2. Instantaneous and progressive healing

HEALING CAN BE
INSTANTANEOUS OR PROGRESSIVE

I want to make known the fact that some healings are instantaneous while others can be progressive. Healing can take place in an instant, within the hour within a day or days. In some cases when Jesus prayed for the sick, the scriptures say that they were healed " that same hour". In other cases, healing may not be manifest for a while.

" And he took the blind man by the hand, and led him out of the town; and when he had spit on his eyes, and put his hands on him, he asked him if he see ought.

And he looked up, and said, I see men as trees, walking.

After he had put his hands again upon his eyes, and made him look up: and he was restored, and saw every man clearly" .
Mark 8:23-25

This is a vivid case of progressive healing. The man's eyes were not perfectly restored when Jesus first prayed for him. Jesus had to pray the second time for him to be perfectly healed. Progressive healing can demand more than one time prayer.

Some Reasons Why Healing Can Be Progressive Are:

1. Imperfect faith - If we waver in our faith our healing my delay until our faith becomes perfected

2. Insufficient anointing - sometimes it takes us spending time with God in prayer and fasting to gain more anointing to minister to the sick. Jesus when His disciples questioned Him concerning the epileptic boy they could not cure, he gave them the answer that " *this kind goeth not out but by prayer and fasting*"

3. The situation might also need deliverance ministration if a demon is involved. Some healing might delay if we are ministering for healing other than for deliverance.If a demon is

involved in that sickness say (a spirit of infirmity) the demon when addressed would leave
and the person's healing would manifest when
healing is prayed for.

4. The sovereign act of God - we many time don't
know why some other healings delay. We can
count it as the sovereign act of God and many
times when the healing comes, God receives
more glory as in the case of Lazarus being dead
for four days.

Preventive Or Relieving Medicine - Choose

Whatever is your case keep on believing God, because
He can heal all your disease. I also want to bring to your
knowledge that the word is medicine to our bodies. We
need to be meditating on God's word concerning our
health before sickness strikes. If sickness tries to invade
a body that has the word, it will not prevail because the
word would act as an anti-body against that sickness,
just like when you get vaccinated against a disease.

If you don't take the word into your life every day as
a means of preventive medicine, you stand a chance of
being attacked by sickness and disease.

By the time you begin to believe in God for your healing after sickness strikes, it can take some time for your
healing to come. It is like when you take medicine to
relieve you of pain, you are not relived immediately; it

takes time for the medicine to work.

> *" My son, attend to my words; incline thine ear unto my sayings,*
>
> *Let them not depart from thine eyes; keep them in the midst of thine heart.*
>
> *For they are life to those that find them, and health (medicine) to all their flesh" .*
>
> *Proverbs 4:20-22*

Desire an essential ingredient

The other thing I believe is worth mentioning concerning our healing is the aspect of desire. The scripture says that if we desire a thing it shall come to pass.

> *" What things soever ye DESIRE, when ye pray, believe that ye receive them, (whatsoever you desire) and ye shall have them (what things so ever you desire)" .*
>
> *Mark 11:24*
>
> *The Bible also warns that " hope deferred maketh the heart sick: but when the DESIRE COMETH it is a tree of life" .*
>
> *Proverbs 13:12*

Desire your healing and you will speedily receive it in

Jesus' name. How much desire have you got to be healed? In other words, do you desire enough to be healed? Your undying desire would speed up your healing process. Do not push your healing for tomorrow receive it today for hope deferred would make your heart sick but when the desire cometh it is a tree of life. Your desire is a tree of life to you.

Procrastination, discouragement and self-pity won't do. Desire to be healed and you would be healed in Jesus' name. You don't have time now to be wallowing in self-pity when you have all the time to walk in divine healing and health.

—Section III—

How To Keep
Your Healing

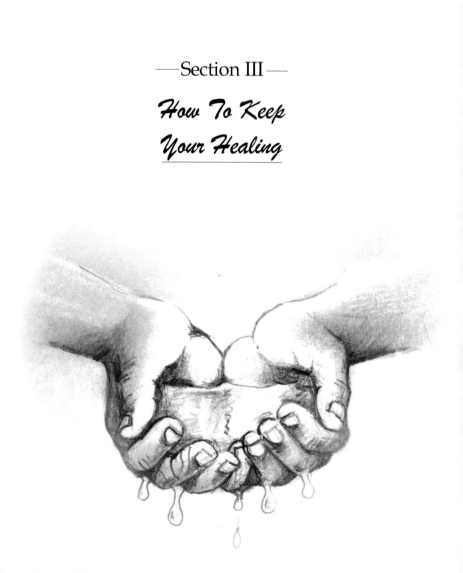

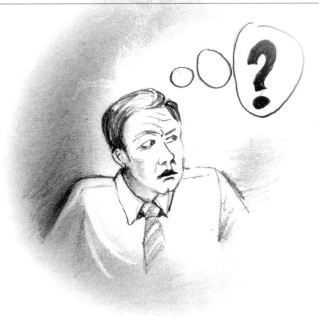

1. *Beware Of Unbelief*

FAITH COMES BY HEARING
NOT BY HAVING HEARD

The scriptures tell us that " faith comes by hearing" and not by having heard. Hearing - is in the present continuous tense, not in the past tense. Many people lose their healing because somewhere along the line they stopped believing God and fall into the trap of unbelief. You have to keep believing God for healing and health for you to walk in health twenty-four seven. The Devil might bring one attack after another but whenever he comes he must meet you believing and prepared for him.

Do not fall into the temptation of encouraging the suggestions of the devil denying the fact that you are healed. If you do you may fall back into sickness once more. It is the same as when believers fall into the trap of the devil and start believing that their Holy Ghost baptism experience was not real. After their experience, they might have listened to someone who told them that speaking in tongue is of the devil. Gradually, unbelief steps in and they stop speaking in tongues. Believe God for your healing and do not encourage unbelief and evil thoughts intending to get you away from the truth.

Emotion or Reality?

In keeping your healing, you need to beware of unbelief. Do not encourage the devil's suggestion that the healing you've experienced was just an emotional thing. Do not let him tell you if you start walking without your crutches you are going to make your condition worse. Believe the report of the LORD. By His stripes you were healed. If you are confident that you were healed, you are healed.

Another thing that causes unbelief is symptoms. Symptoms can also cause your faith to be short lived. Believe the word of God instead of the symptoms. Symptoms can be deceiving. Also if you are confident of your healing especially in areas of your body you cannot verify from the outside, go to your doctor and let them run another test to verify your healing, you will see the result of your faith when the test verifies your healing.

Faith is a Walk and a fight

Faith is a walk. It is a walk in the midst of troubling circumstances, but having done all, we can stand. Stand, therefore, and be strong in your faith. We all when we were babies learned to walk. In the Spirit we also need to learn to walk by faith. Through faith and patience you will obtain your promise.

" *That ye be not slothful, but followers of them who through faith and patience obtain the promises*"

Hebrew 6:12

" *(For we walk of faith; and not by sight:)*"

2Corinthians 5:7

Faith is a fight. Praise the LORD it is a good fight. Fight the good fight of faith, resist the devil and he will flee from you. Cast down every thought and imagination that seeks to exalt itself above the knowledge you have of God healing you. Speak to them; tell them to be obedient to the word of God.

" Fight the good fight of faith, lay hold on eternal life, whereunto thou art also called, and hast confessed a good profession before many witnesses "

2Timothy 6:12

To lay hold on eternal living (health) we need to fight the fight of faith. It is a good fight though because the battle has been won for us when He confessed that it is all finished for us, on the cross of Calvary. Have you confessed your healing before many witnesses? Then you have made a good confession. Now your calling into healing is made sure by your confession - you are healed.

Come!

" And Peter answered him and said, Lord, if it be thou, bid me come unto thee in the water.

And he said, come. And when Peter was come down out of the ship, he walked on the water, to go to Jesus.

But when he saw the wind boisterous, he was afraid; and beginning to sink, he cried, saying, Lord, save me.

And immediately Jesus stretched forth his hand, and caught him, and said unto him, O thou of little faith, wherefore didst thou doubt?

Matthew 14:28-31

This is the account of when Peter saw Jesus walking on the water. He too wanted to walk on the water. Jesus bade him " come ". Peter began to walk on the water as he took heed to the word " come ". Immediately he stopped believing the word for fear of the storm, he began to sink. Doubts and unbelief can cause you to sink down into trouble. DON'T DOUBT.

When Peter was walking on the water, it was as natural for him as if he was walking on dry land. Faith is the natural walk of the believer. But when Peter took his eyes off faith, it was disastrous for him. Another thing I want to bring to your notice is that the storm and wind were there at the beginning when Peter started walking on the water.

He might not have recognised the storm when he first started walking on the water because of his faith, but the storm did not stop him walking in the water. He was doing all right. It was when he began to be mindful of the storm at the expense of Jesus' word " come " that he began to sink. Fight the good fight of faith. Victory is yours in Jesus' name. Do not consider the storm consider the word of God.

" And being not weak in faith, he considered not his own body now dead when he was about an hundred years old, neither yet the deadness of Sarah's womb:

He staggered not at the promise of God through unbelief; but was strong in faith, giving glory to God;

And being fully persuaded that, what he hath promised, he is able also to perform. "

Romans 4:19-21

In your fight of faith you do not consider the problem. It is not that you deny the presence of the problem no! It is that you deny the power of the problem as you compare it to the authority of the word of God. Like in this story, Abraham had three problems. The first one was that he was too old to bare a child; Sarah his wife also was barren and also too old to bare a child. Abraham knew that but he just would not consider it.

He staggered not at the promise of God. People with strong faith would not doubt God's word. People with strong faith would even start to give God glory and praise for healing them because they are fully persuaded that what God has promised He is also able to perform.

If you are fully persuaded of the promise of God there is going to be a performance on your account.

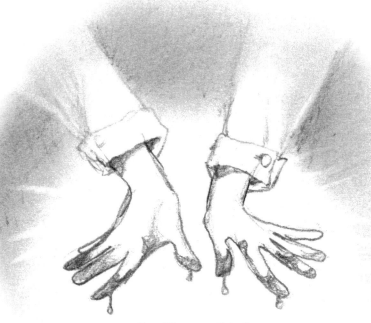

2. Beware Of Sin

SIN NO MORE LEST A
WORSE THING COME ON YOU

" *There was a certain man there, which had an infirmity thirty and eight years.*

And Jesus saith unto him, Rise, take up thy bed, and walk.

Afterwards Jesus findeth him in the temple, and said unto him, Behold, thou art made whole: SIN NO MORE, LEST A WORSE THING COME UNTO THEE"

John 5:5,8,14

This man was sick for thirty-eight years. The reason for his infirmity was because of his sin. We were not told what his sin was but we were made to understand that his sin brought about his sickness. Jesus knew that his sin caused his sickness and yet Jesus healed him. I don't know why Jesus did not point out his sin to him before praying for him. Maybe it would have hindered his faith by putting heavy guilt on him, I don't know.

Maybe Jesus had seen that he had suffered enough and did not want his sins before his eyes at this time. All the same, AFTERWARDS Jesus FOUND him in the temple and said to him, SIN NO MORE, LEST A WORSE THING COME UNTO THEE.

We also see a similar situation in the book of James:

" Is anyone sick among you? let him call for the elders of the Church; and let them pray over him, anointing him with oil in the name of the Lord:

And the prayer of faith shall save the sick, and the Lord shall raise him up; and if he have committed sins, they shall be forgiven him.

Confess your faults one to another, and pray one for another, that ye may be healed. The effectual fervent prayer of a righteous man availeth much."

James 5:14-16

I don't know why confessing sins came after the prayers but we know that whether the sins is confessed before or after the healing God does forgive and healing does take place.

Sin caused this man to be sick, and sin could cause a worse sickness to come upon him. Sin must not be tolerated. It is an enemy not a friend. Maybe your cancer came upon you because of your bad smoking habit, or that liver problem came because you drink too much alcohol. Your blood disease might have come through your promiscuous sex life. Now that you are healed, the Lord is saying, sin no more because a worse thing can come into your life as a result.

Maybe your sickness is as a result of a demonic attack. Some sicknesses are as result of a demonic attack - a spirit of infirmity. When that demon is cast out and you are delivered, you had better accept Jesus as your Saviour and Lord and keep away from sin lest seven more demons come upon you. Your last state will be worse than the first. So therefore do not accept sin.

" When an unclean spirit is gone out of a man, he walketh through dry places, seeking rest, and findeth none.

Then he saith, I will return to my house from whence I came out; and when he is come, he findeth it empty, swept and garnished.

Then goeth he, and taketh with himself seven other spirits more wicked than himself, and they enter in and dwell there: and the last state of that man is worse than the first..."

Matthew 12:43-45

Sin gives occasion for the devil to take advantage of us. Sin breaks the covenant for God's protection from sickness in our lives. The Bible still warns that the wages of sin is death so keep away from death.

" *For the wages of sin is death...*"

Romans 3:23

" *...And sin, when it is finished, bringeth forth death*"

James 1:15

Unforgiveness

The sin of an unforgiving heart also hinders the healing of many. It can prevent you from being healed and cause you to shrink back into sickness and disease. An unforgiving heart exposes you to demonic torments and demonic afflictions. An unforgiving heart can open the door to sicknesses like cancer and arthritis in your life. The God who heals will not tolerate an unforgiving heart. He will not even hear your prayers if you are unforgiving in

your heart. Forgive who ever have sinned against you and
God will forgive, heal and sustain you.

> " *And when you stand praying, forgive, if you have
> ought against any: that your Father also which is in
> heaven may forgive you your trespasses.*
>
> *But if you do not forgive, neither will your Father which
> is in heaven forgive your trespasses"*
>
> *Mark 11:25-26*
>
> " *And his lord was wroth, and delivered him to the tor-
> mentors, till he should pay all that was due unto him.*
>
> *So likewise shall my heavenly Father do also unto you,
> if ye from your hearts forgive not every one his brother
> thier trespasses.*"
>
> *Matthew 18:34-35*

This servant was forgiven. He refused to forgive
his fellow servant, so he was handed over to
tormentors (demons) till he could pay his debt. If
you allow grudge, hate and unforgiveness in your
heart, your healing will not stay, so drop it and
stay healed.

——— Section 4 ———

How To
Administer Healing

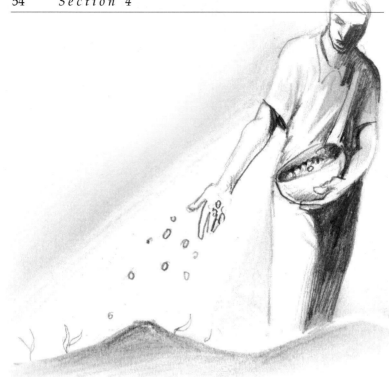

1. *Go And Preach*

THE GOSPEL OF JESUS
IS A HEALING GOSPEL

*"And he said unto them, GO YE INTO ALL THE WORLD,
AND PREACH THE GOSPEL to every creature.*

*He that believeth and is baptised shall be saved; but he that
believeth not shall be damned.*

*And these signs shall follow them that believe; in my name
they shall cast out devils; they shall speak with new
tongues;*

They shall take up serpents; and if they drink any deadly thing, it shall not hurt them; THEY SHALL LAY HANDS ON THE SICK AND THEY SHALL RECOVER.

And they went forth, and preached everywhere, THE LORD WORKING WITH THEM, AND CONFIRMING THE WORD WITH SIGNS FOLLOWING. AMEN.

Mark 16:15-18,20

The Lord commissioned His disciples (that includes us) to go into the whole world and preach the Gospel to every creature. There are a few things I want to highlight concerning these verses of scripture. The first is that we need to GO and PREACH. If we don't go, it is obvious that the Lord will not have anyone to go with. If we don't preach, there is nothing for Him to confirm. Secondly, we are to preach the Gospel. The gospel is good news. The Gospel is:

" *How God anointed Jesus Christ of Nazareth with the Holy Ghost and with power: who went about doing good, and healing all that were oppressed of the devil; for God was with Him* ".

Acts12: 38

Whenever we preach the healing gospel, people will have faith to be healed. That is the purpose of this book that is why I preach or teach the healing Gospel. I want people to be healed of whatever sickness and disease they have plaguing them. If you are going to a Church that does not preach about God wanting to heal you, you will not know what to do in times of sickness and you won't stand any chance of overcoming it. I Pray ignorance do not take you to an early grave. Many loving believers have died of sicknesses and diseases because of ignorance. Do not add to the number!

Them that believe

" *And these signs shall follow them that believe ...*"

Mark 16:15

These signs shall follow THEM THAT BELIEVE. It did not say they shall only follow the Pastor, or Evangelist, but " them that believe" . Any one who has faith enough to preach it shall lay their hands on the sick and they shall recover. Husband; lay your hand on your sick wife! Wife, do likewise! Parent, will you dare believe God for your sick child? Child, will you believe God for your dying mother?

If you will dare to believe, then start preaching that God wants to heal that loved one, lay your hands on that sick person and pray, then leave the other aspect, " and they shall recover" , to God. It is none of your business! Do not worry yourself about how they shall recover, that is God's business not yours.

Many people ask the question about why people are not healed and so on. Well many have not heard the healing gospel enough and "how can they hear without a preacher?" Many also have not believed because they have no faith to be healed. The more we preach the healing gospel the more people will have faith to be healed and they would be healed.

The Lord will confirm His word

" And they went forth, and preached every where, AND THE LORD WORKING WITH THEM, AND CON-FIRMING THE WORD WITH SIGNS FOLLOWING"

Mark 16:20

The world today is being afflicted with sickness and diseases because there are not enough people out there who will dare to preach and pray for the sick. People don't believe in divine healing anymore, it has been labelled as a thing of the past because we don't hear it preached any more. If you will dare to preach, God will do the signs and the wonders.

" LONG TIME therefore abode they speaking boldly in the Lord, WHICH GAVE TESTIMONY, unto the

word of his grace, and granted SIGNS and WONDERS to be done by their hands".

Acts 14:3

The apostles would not have had many sick people healed in Iconium if they had not remained there a long time preaching with boldness that God wanted to heal them. The Lord would not have given testimony and caused the miracles to happen if they had not preached.

" And there they preached the gospel.

And there sat a certain man at Lystra, impotent in his feet, being a cripple from his mother's womb, who never had walked:

And the same HEARD PAUL SPEAK: who steadfast-ly beholding him, AND PERCEIVING THAT HE HAD FAITH TO BE HEALED.

Said with a loud voice, stand upright on thy feet. And he leaped and walked".

Acts 14:7-10

The very first step to minister healing to the sick is to go and preach the healing Gospel. We need to hear more healing messages in our crusades, seminars and Church conventions today. Faith will then develop in the hearts of the people and the Lord will honour their faith with His healing power in Jesus' name.

No one can tell me that sickness and disease is not an issue in the world we live in today. It is a major issue like it was in Jesus' days. And if Jesus had to get Himself involved in solving that problem for His generation can't we tap into that same anointing and help in our own generation?

" *And Jesus went about all Galilee, teaching in their synagogues, and preaching the gospel of the kingdom, and healing all manner of sickness and all manner of disease among the people.*

And his fame went throughout Syria; and they brought unto him all sick people that were taken with diverse diseases and torments, and those who were possessed with devils, and those who were lunatick, and those who had the palsy; and he healed them"

Matthew 4:23-24

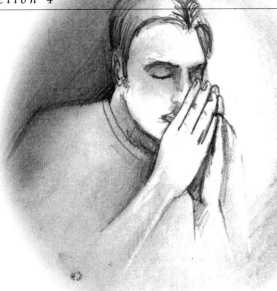

2. *The Prayer Of Faith*

THE PRAYER OF FAITH
WILL SAVE THE SICK

" Is any sick among you? Let him call for the elders of the Church; and let them pray over him ...

AND THE PRAYER OF FAITH shall save the sick, and the Lord shall raise him up; and if he had committed sins, they shall be forgiven him" .

James 5:14-15

James here is asking if anyone is sick among the followers of Christ. Sickness should not necessarily be a problem among them but should there be a case or two, this is what he advised them to do. " Let him CALL for the elders of the Church" . The elders will come and say a prayer in faith for him and the PRAYER SAID IN FAITH WILL SAVE HIM (make him well). If the sickness were as a result of his sins, his sins would be forgiven him as he confesses them.

" Confess your faults one to another, and pray for one another, that ye may be healed. The effectual fervent prayer of a righteous man availeth much".

James 5:16

Many believers today make the issue of sin prevent them from praying for a sick brother or sister. Our attitude is like " let him stew in his own juice for a while; it is God teaching him a lesson ". We become judgmental rather than being compassionate. The Bible says that if he has committed sins, they shall be forgiven him if he confesses them.

God is not faultfinding. Any sins confessed He forgives. He will not hold anything against you. He has sent Jesus to pay the price for sins. Stop being self-righteous and stop sinking into self-pity and " make straight paths for your feet, lest that which is lame be taken out of the way" .

The prayer said with fervent faith by righteous elders in accordance with God's word is effective in its working. The prayer of faith will save the sick and forgive his sins.

The prayer of faith is an antidote to sickness and disease. It carries no "if" , no " maybe " and no " what if " with it. It just saves the sick and makes them whole again. It is a " thus says the Lord" , so there is no need to ask God if it is His will. It is God's will to heal the sick.

Speak to the sickness and tell it to leave according to *Mark 11:22-23*. Cast it out, and it will leave. Shout the shout of victory and let the glory fall. The Lord will then heal the sick and all will be well.

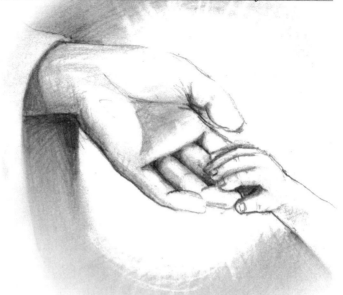

3. Pray To The Father In Jesus Name

ASK THE FATHER
IN MY NAME

" And in that day ye shall ask me nothing. Verily verily I say unto you, whatsoever ye shall ASK THE FATHER IN MY NAME, he will give it you.

Hitherto have ye asked nothing in my name: ask, and ye shall receive, that your joy may be full.

For the Father himself loveth you, because ye have loved me, and have believed that I have come out from God "

John 16:23, 24, 27

Jesus was talking here about after His death and resurrection. Plainly speaking, He was talking about today. Jesus' disciples have been asking Him for everything. They asked Him for food for the hungry, healing for the sick etc. Jesus knew that His earthly ministry would soon be over. He would not be available to be asked to do anything else for them, so He was preparing them for that day.

Jesus was establishing a principle, which His disciples would be able to use on that day. That principle is " asking the Father in Jesus name." Jesus also wants to express the fact that He is here to do the Father's will, and that His willingness to do things for His disciples is a total act of surrender to God's will. No wonder Jesus said, "For the Father himself loves you."

Jesus now stands at the right hand of the Father making intercession for us. When we approach the Father in Jesus' name, His blood speaks for us and God will remember His covenant which He has signed for us. The name and blood of Jesus then acts as a key to unlock His heavenly blessings for us.

Jesus also knows the grief and sorrow we feel when we are sick, he wants our joy to be full. No wonder he bore all our grief and carried all our sorrows. Ask for your healing that your joy may be full.

> " *Verily, verily I say unto you, he that believeth on me, the works that I do shall he do also; and greater works than these shall he do; because I go unto my father.*

*And whatsoever ye shall ask in my name, that will I do,
that the father may be glorified in the son.*

If ye shall ask anything in my name, I will do it" .

John 14:12-14

In John chapter 16, Jesus was talking about prayer in
the sense of petition, supplication and requests.
However, in John 14, He is talking about taking your
stand in His name, demanding what is yours from the
hands of the adversary. Jesus here is talking about doing
the works. Sickness and disease will flee at the mention
of the name of Jesus; they can't resist that name.

Use the name of Jesus against any adversary and that
adversary will bow at the mention of His name. They
recognise the Lordship of the name of Jesus and they will
bow at the mention of His majestic name.

*" Wherefore God has highly exalted him, and given him
a name which is above every name:*

*That at the name of Jesus every knee should bow, of
thing in Heaven, and things in Earth, and things under
the earth;*

*And that every tongue should confess that Jesus Christ
is Lord, to the glory of God the father.*

Philippians 2:9-11

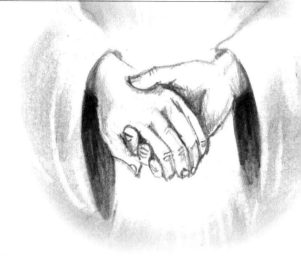

4. Prayer Of Intercession

THE SPIRIT HELPS
IN OUR INFIRMITIES

" Likewise the Spirit also helpeth our infirmities: for we know not what we should pray for as we ought: but the Spirit itself maketh intercession for us with groaning which cannot be uttered.

And he that searcheth the hearts knoweth what is the mind of the Spirit, because he maketh intercession for the saints according to the will of God" .
Romans 8:26-27

The Spirit of God always helps us in our infirmities. In some cases when dealing with sickness and diseases, we have little or no result. In such cases we need to spend time in intercession for the person. In relying on the Holy Spirit, He can then give us vital information that is relevant to the person's healing and deliverance.

In some cases, the sickness may have been caused by demons. Ordinarily ministering for healing will not bring about much result in the life of the person, but casting out the demon will. Some other cases are as a result of ancestral or self-imposed curses. In such cases, the curses need to be broken. In some other cases, the Holy Spirit may witness to you when interceding that the person has an unforgiving heart. The Spirit also helps our infirmities (weaknesses and short comings) as we make intercessions for the sick.

Through intercession you share in the person's sufferings, as Christ also has suffered for you. By that I mean you are able to identify with the person's need and feel the way he feels. Through identifying yourself with the person's infirmity you are able to pray through with compassion for him to get well.

Sickness is an infirmity. The Holy Spirit helps not only in the area of praying, but also in the area of recovery. By praying in the Holy Ghost, we inspire and build up our faith, thus building our substance or energy to bring about the desired healing. The Spirit then releases that energy upon the sick and heals them.

" But ye, beloved, building up yourselves on your most holy faith, praying in the Holy Ghost"

Jude 20

We cannot get anyone healed without faith and the anoiting of the Holy spirit. So rely on the Holy Spirit for healing to be made manifest.

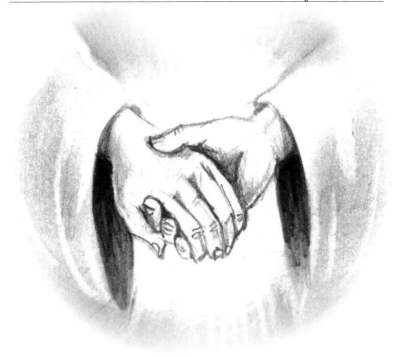

5. *Prayer Of Agreement*

AGREE IN
HIS NAME

" Again I say unto you, that if two of you shall agree on earth as touching any thing that they shall ask, it shall be done for them of my father which is in heaven.

For where two or three are gathered together in my name, there am I in the midst of them "

Matthew 18:19-20

The prayer of agreement is a powerful weapon against sickness and diseases. It brings together corporate anointing and corporate faith against the power of sickness and disease. This is vital on many occasions for healing to take place.

It is good to ask the congregation regularly to join their faith with yours when you are praying for the sick. If other ministers are there, that is also a blessing. With all these people gathered in the name of Jesus, there are bound to be miracles. Get every unbelieving person out of that room like Jesus did at Jairus' place and pray with people with like precious faith and the prayer of agreement will save the sick. When there is one accord in one place there is bound to be miracles.

" *And Peter, fastening his eyes upon him with John, said, LOOK ON US,*

And HE GAVE HEED UNTO THEM EXPECTING to receive something of them.

Then Peter said, Silver and gold have I none; but such as I have give I thee: In the name of Jesus Christ of Nazareth rise up and walk.

And he took him by the right hand, and lifted him up: and immediately his feet and ankle bones received strength"

Acts 3:4-7

Peter said to the man " look on us" . There was agreement there. The man looked "on them expecting to receive something from them". Peter gave the command, the anointing was so strong on Peter that he could not help but lift the man up. It was completed, the man's anklebones received strength and he was healed.

We have seen many miracles happen as we agree together in faith for the sick to be healed. His word is effective and His principles works. Heaven and earth would pass away but His word abides forever.

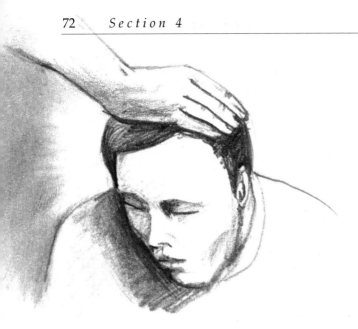

6. *Laying On Of Hands*

LAY HANDS
ON THE SICK

" *... They shall lay their hands on the sick, and they shall recover".*

Mark 16:18

The Church has no problem in taking the Gospel to the entire World. Praise the Lord. This is wonderful. It is vision-based and I love it. I am also praying that the same vision will be directed towards healing the sick.

We find taking the Gospel to the world and healing the sick in the same context in scripture. Jesus preached the Gospel and healed the sick. The one who saves the sinner is the same one who heals the sick. So in taking the Gospel to the sinner, lay hands on the sick that they may recover.

The doctrine of laying on of hands is a biblical ordinance to impart healing, blessing and authority. Through the act of laying on of hands, we exercise authority against sickness in the name of Jesus and anointing and faith is released to heal the sick.

Sometimes the person being prayed for actually feels the release of power in a warm or cold air coming on them or like an electric shock in their body. Sometimes nothing is felt at all, the person only observes that the sickness or disease has left them. Your hands are a point of contact to transmit healing to the sick. So what are you waiting for? Lay your hands on the sick and they shall recover.

7. *Anointing With Oil In Faith*

ANOINT THE
SICK WITH OIL

" *Is any sick among you? Let him call for the elders of the Church; and let them pray over him, ANOINTING HIM WITH OIL IN THE NAME OF THE LORD:*

And the prayer of faith shall save the sick, and the Lord shall raise him up; and if he have committed sins, they shall be forgiven him " .

James 5:14-15

Another way we should minister to the sick is by the anointing oil. We observe that the prayer of faith and the name of Jesus should accompany anointing with oil. It is like taking a pill with a glass of water, or like the different components of the pills you take.

Oil is a symbol of the Holy Ghost. It represents the anointing released for healing on the sick. The prayer of faith said in the name of the Lord (when oil is poured on the sick) will save him from his sickness. That anointing removes burdens and destroys yokes. That released anointing, according to James, also forgives sins. Praise the Lord!

" When Jesus saw their faith, he said to the sick of the palsy, son, THY SINS BE FORGIVEN YOU "

Mark 2:5

" And it shall come to pass in that day, that HIS BUR-DEN shall be taken away from off thy shoulder, and HIS YOKE from off thy neck, and the yoke shall be destroyed BECAUSE OF THE ANOINTING"

Isaiah 10:27

The devil's yokes and burdens (sicknesses and diseases) are taken and destroyed by the anointing of the

Holy Ghost and our healing is made complete. We will talk about the healing anointing in the next chapter.

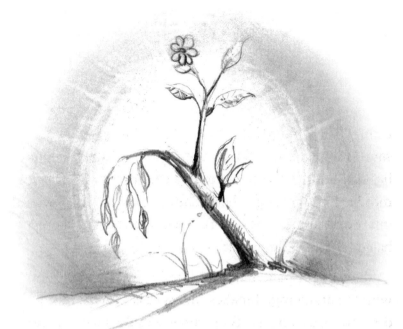

8. The Gifts of Healing(s)

HEALING ANOINTING

" *To another faith by the same Spirit; to another the gifts of healing by the same Spirit;*"

1Corinthians 12:9

This gift of the Spirit called " the gifts of healing" in Greek really should be the gift(s) of healing(s). It is more than one gift and there is more than just one kind of healing.

Some ministers are more anointed to get people healed from one kind of disease than another. Some ministers have got the gift of healing people with cancer whilst others get many people in wheel chairs healed.

Other ministers have got two, three or four gifts of healing. The anointing is different, but ministered by the same Holy Spirit. Some ministers get more people healed through the anointing cloth whereas others get more healing through their shadow touching people as in the case of the apostles. Yet other ministers get people healed by punching them.

We can get people healed by the prayer of faith but with the anointing, it makes things easier. It gets the job done twice as quickly. Sometimes you do not even pray for people, the Holy Spirit starts healing them all over the place as the word is preached or when people start praising and worshipping God.

We ministers need to pray that the Spirit of the Lord be present to heal in our services. It is a wonderful experience.

Points Of Contact

" And by the hands of the apostles were many mighty signs and wonders wrought among the people...

And believers were the more added to the Lord, multitudes both of men and women.)

Insomuch that they brought forth the sick into the streets, and laid them on beds and couches, that at the least the shadow of Peter passing by might overshadow some of them"

Acts 5:12,14,15

Healing anointing could be transferred through points of contact. By points of contact we mean material things like clothes, aprons, handkerchiefs, and even through a believer's shadow.

We see anointing coming out of Jesus' clothes in the healing of the woman with the issue of blood. We also see Peter's shadow as a point of contact healing the multitudes in the streets.

" And God wrought special miracles by the hands of Paul:

So that from his body were brought unto the sick handkerchiefs or aprons, and the diseases departed from them, and the evil spirits went out of them"

Acts 19:11-12

Here we see handkerchiefs and aprons as points of contact transferring anointing for healing and deliverance for the sick and oppressed. There is no limit to the power of God made available towards the sick. The methods God has for healing the sick are vast; so open up to receive from Him.

The more believers seek the face of God for their healing, the more God will heal the sick. When God begins to heal the sick, the more people's faith will be strengthened and we will never know what people's faith will tell them to do. When they obey; God will honour their faith. The Bible did not say the Apostles told them to do what they did. The boldness of their faith told them to do what they did.

Our faith in the anointing to come would bring our deliverance sooner and in greater proportion than we would ever imagine. We are yet to see more outstanding healing and miracle than we now see in our day.

Proxy Prayers

In areas directed by the Holy Ghost, proxy prayer can be made for loved ones who cannot be present at the place of prayers due to distance and other related problems.

If the Holy Spirit directs it, the relation standing in proxy for the sick sometimes goes through all the manifestations of the sick person. At the same time God will also be moving in the life of the sick or demon afflicted person, bringing healing and deliverance to them.

We also see that aprons and handkerchiefs were taken from the body of Paul and used to pray for the sick and to cast out demons. This I believe was done to get healed those who cannot get to the place of meeting.

" *And God wrought special miracles by the hands of Paul:*

So that from his body were brought to the sick handkerchiefs, or aprons, and the diseases departed from them, and the evil spirits went out of them"

Acts 19:11-12

—— Section V ——

*According
To Your Faith*

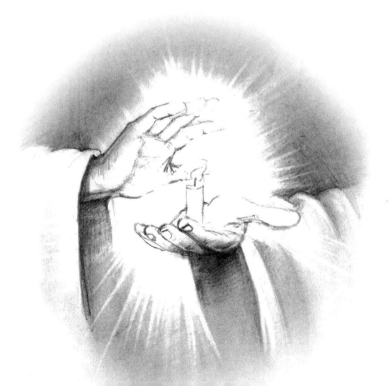

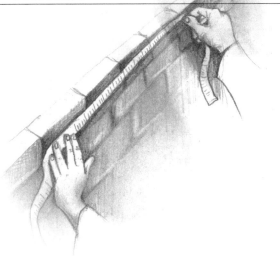

1. *According To Your Faith*

THE MEASURE
YOU MEASURE

We all believe in a measure. In other words we all have a measure of faith. God gave us all the measure of faith when we got born again however; we need to grow in faith. If faith can be measured how much faith have you got?

" ...*According as God hath dealt to every man the measure of faith*"

Romans 12:3

This measure can grow depending on the measure of the Word of God we meditate upon. We can allow the measure of the word of God in us to drop if we fail to meditate on the word of God.

> " And he said unto them, Take heed what ye hear: the measure ye mete, it shall be measured unto you: and unto you that hear shall more be given
>
> For he that hath, to him shall be given: and he that hath not, from him shall be taken even that which he hath"
>
> Mark 4:24-25

The one who has the word of healing stored up in him will have health in abundance, the one who does not have the word of healing stored up in him might be in health at the moment, but his health will be taken away from him if sickness strikes because he has nothing to stop it with. How much measure of faith are you willing and ready to put for your healing to take place?

Our faith's growth depends on our meditation level. What we have stored up in us through meditation we confess, and what we confess we act upon. Our confession is the groundwork for God to act on our behalf. To have the faith of God we need to meditate on the word of God through which we can receive anything from God.

One person's faith may grow more than another's depending on the measure of the word of God stored up in them. The-woman-with-the issue-of-blood's faith was greater than that of Jairus' and the Centurion's faith was so great that Jesus commended him for his great faith.

You can start believing God where you are at the moment and the more you continue meditating on the word of God the more your faith will grow. Nothing is impossible to those who believe. You can start believing God for a successful operation. You can go on to believe God for no operation at all for your healing depending on the measure you measure.

Many people don't receive their healing because they have been asked to believe on a level their faith has not reached. You know at what level your faith is. Get someone to believe with you on that level and you will be healed as you have imagined it.

What Would You That I Should Do?

" And Jesus answered and said unto him, what would thou that I should do unto thee? The blind man said unto him, Lord, that I might receive my sight"

Mark 10:51

Jesus always asks those who come to Him for help what they want him to do for them. He always does as

He is asked. Jairus asked Him to come and lay His hands on his child, and that He did. The Centurion asked Him to " speak the word only" that He did. It is always good for us to know what we want God to do for us and tell Him so when we want Him to heal us. The method by which we ae healed is determined by what we ask in prayer.

You can receive your healing by laying on of hands; you can believe God for a successful operation or divine surgery. It is what YOU would have Him to do he would do. Would you have the preacher anoint you or do you want him to speak the word only? The preacher can encourage you to believe at a greater level of faith, but it is up to you to believe at the level you are able. However, when God begins to show Himself strongly on your behalf, you will begin to believe Him to a greater level.

" Therefore I say unto you, what things so ever you desire when you pray, believe that you receive them and you shall have them"

Mark 11:24

It is what you desire you ask for in prayer. " What would you have me do" should be " what thing so ever you desire" . And if you believe that you receive them, you shall have them.

According To Your Faith
So Be It Unto You

" Then touched he their eyes, saying, According to your faith be it unto you"

Matthew 9:29

There are people who say: " if God wants to heal me, why doesn't He just go ahead and do so" ? " Why do I have to believe him to heal me" ? Well, why did Jesus ask the two blind men what they wanted when He knew they were blind? Everyone could see Bartimaeus was blind. Why did Jesus ask what he wanted? God does not impose Himself on anybody. By telling Him what you want you are establishing two things:

1.   That you are giving Him the invitation to work on your behalf.

2.   That you have faith to be healed.

These are two things we need to consider because they are vital for our healing to take place. Know what you want God to do for you and ask Him just that. According to your faith it will be unto you.

God is a faith God. He would like us to act in faith too. " Call the things, which be not as though they were", and they would be yours in Jesus' name.

Jesus the Healer

Jesus is our healer. His healing ministry was very unique and very powerful. He never lost a patient He healed them all. Why was His healing ministry so unique? What can we learn from Him to make our own healing ministry unique and powerful? Here are a few things I have gathered from Jesus' ministry, which I believe, can be of help to us.

It was written about Him

And there was delivered unto him the book of the prophet Esaias. And when he had opened the book, he found the place where it was written,

The Spirit of the Lord is upon me, because he hath anointed me to preach the gospel to the poor; he hath sent me to heal the brokenhearted, to preach deliverance to the captives, and recovering of sight to the blind, to set at liberty them that are bruised,

To preach the acceptable year of the Lord.

And he closed the book, and he gave it again to the minister, and sat down. And the eyes of all them that were in the synagogue were fastened on him.

And he began to say unto them, This day is this scripture fulfilled in your ears.

And all bare him witness, and wondered at the gracious

words which proceeded out of his mouth. And they said,
Is not this Joseph's son?

And he said unto them, Ye will surely say unto me this
proverb, Physician, heal thyself: whatsoever we have
heard done in Capernaum, do also here in thy country.

Luke 4:17-23

It was written of Him that He would heal. Jesus
found the place where it was written of him that He
would heal, read it and closed the chapter - He fulfilled
it. If we are to heal the sick we need to find out whether
it is written in Scriptures that we can do just that. I
believe this is not a problem at this time now because we
have found out from numerous scriptures that it is written about us to heal the sick.

Anointed to Heal

" *How God anointed Jesus of Nazareth with the Holy*
Ghost and with power: who went about doing good, and
healing all that were oppressed of the devil; for God was
with him."

We can do nothing without God. Jesus was anointed
(empowered) to heal when the Spirit of God came upon
Him at His baptism. Jesus never did any healing or miracle before that time. We know that because the scrip-

ture tells us that the first miracle Jesus ever did was to turn water into wine.

" This beginning of miracles did Jesus in Cana of Galilee, and manifested forth his glory; and his disciples believed on him."

John 2:11

Are we anointed to heal? We have been anointed and given authority By Jesus Christ who has all authority in heaven and on earth to heal the sick. As the Father sent Jesus even so has He sent us. The works of healing which He did shall we do also and greater healing works we will do He has promised.

" And as ye go, preach, saying, The kingdom of heaven is at hand.

Heal the sick, cleanse the lepers, raise the dead, cast out devils: freely ye have received, freely give."

Matthew 10:7-8

" To another faith by the same Spirit; to another the gifts of healing by the same Spirit."

1Corinthians 12:9

Jesus had the gifts of healings. He was anointed by God to heal and God was with Him when He healed the sick. We as Christians must pray for the anointing to heal the sick and for God to be with us while we are doing it. We need the manifest presence of God with us to heal the sick. The previous scripture said that God was with Jesus and Jesus also promised us that:

" And they went forth, and preached every where, the Lord working with them, and confirming the word with signs following. Amen."

Mark 16:20

When God's presence is made manifest in our lives, the power of the Lord would be present to heal the sick.

As I hear I judge

" I can of mine own self do nothing: as I hear, I judge: and my judgment is just; because I seek not mine own will, but the will of the Father which hath sent me."

John 5:30

I believe Jesus enquired of God concerning the people He healed. Because He was always in that state of waiting and enquiring from God, God speaks to Him concerning the people who came to Him for healing. The Bible says that He constantly groaned in His Spirit coming to Lazarus' grave. He was enquiring of the Spirit of

God.   As He hears, He is able to judge or discern how that healing must take place. I believe, sometimes Jesus did not only hear from God He also saw in a vision how God wanted to heal the sick.

" *But Jesus answered them, My Father worketh hither-to, and I work.*"

John 5:17

" *Then answered Jesus and said unto them, Verily, ver-ily, I say unto you, The Son can do nothing of himself, BUT WHAT HE SEETH the Father do: for what things soever he doeth, these also doeth the Son likewise.*"
    John 5:19

Do not limit the extent to which God can go to heal the sick.   He loves to heal the sick.   He has not stopped heal-ing the sick at all.   He still does His work - healing the sick and you qualify for that healing because, " by His stripes you were healed."

Jesus went about healing

" *How God anointed Jesus of Nazareth with the Holy*

Ghost and with power: who went about doing good, and healing all that were oppressed of the devil; for God was with him."

If we want healing to take place we need to be in the healing business.

If we don't go out and heal them they won't be healed, would they? What are you waiting for? Go on and pray for that sick one and expect them to recover. Pastor, begin to pray for the sick in your services, expect to hear from God in the process and pray for the anointing to heal and the results would be out of this world.

Not according to the course of the world

" And you hath he quickened, who were dead in trespasses and sins;

Wherein in time past ye walked according to the course of this world, according to the prince of the power of the air, the spirit that now worketh in the children of disobedience:

Among whom also we all had our conversation in times past in the lusts of our flesh, fulfilling the desires of the flesh and of the mind; and were by nature the children of wrath, even as others.

But God, who is rich in mercy, for his great love where-with he loved us,

Even when we were dead in sins, hath quickened us together with Christ, (by grace ye are saved;)

And hath raised us up together, and made us sit together in heavenly places in Christ Jesus:

That in the ages to come he might shew the exceeding riches of his grace in his kindness toward us through Christ Jesus."

Ephesians 2:1-7

The Devil has created a course, a pattern a plan for this world. That course is for the world to walk in sickness and disease. At one point in our lives when we were unsaved, we walked according to that pattern but now we operate at a higher level above sickness and disease. We walk far above that course which is operated by principalities and powers. That was the position where Jesus was operating from.

Jesus gave us authority over sickness and disease and every demon to drive them out in His name. We are seated together with Him in heavenly places with sickness and diseases under us.

When God commissions us to do certain things, He positions us above whatever authority or power He has commissioned us to challenge. When God sent Moses to Egypt he had to make him god to Pharaoh. God also had to give him a prophet in the person of his brother Aaron. Moses' problem was that he saw himself insignificant to his subject so he asked the question, " Who am I to go before Pharaoh" . God was trying to make a god out of Moses and he was seeing himself as nothing.

For Moses to stand against Pharaoh who was god in Egypt, Moses was to be operating on a higher level than that of Pharaoh. For us to drive out demons, plunder hell and destroy the works of the Devil (with sickness being a part of it) we have to operate on a higher level than that of Satan.

" And the Lord said unto Moses, See, I have made thee a god to Pharaoh: and Aaron thy brother shall be thy prophet.

Thou shalt speak all that I command thee: and Aaron thy brother shall speak unto Pharaoh, that he send the children of Israel out of his land."

Exodus 7:1-2

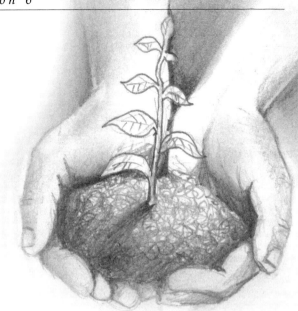

LONGEVITY OF LIFE

This is a very important chapter. It climaxes the rest. If we do not know that it is God's will for us to walk in divine health, we will not be able to understand that He would also like for us to live long on this earth. God's will for us is that we live a long, healthy and wealthy life in this world. A long, satisfying and fulfilled life is our portion on this earth. If we stay healed, then we would live long on this earth won't we?

" Because he hath set his love upon me, therefore will I deliver him: I will set him on high, because he hath known my name.

He shall call upon me, and I will answer him: I will be

with him in trouble; I will deliver him, and honour him. With long life will I satisfy him, and show him my salvation".

Psalm 91:14-16

From this portion of scriptures, we see three pre-requisites for longevity of life. The believer who:

- Set his love upon the Lord
- Know the Lord's name
- And call upon that name

Will be guaranteed (6) things:

- Deliverance from trouble
- Exaltation
- Answer to prayers
- Honour
- Satisfied with long life
- Quality long life

We see from these verses of scriptures that the one who fulfils those three requirements will live a long, full and satisfying life. Quality long life is the full and perfect will of God for every believer.

The purpose of God for our lives is not that we should be killed, or die early in life or to suffer some kind of malady. Many people argue that the Lord can take some believer early in life. They use the phrase, " The Lord took him" . This is a wrong use of scripture. The Bible only mentioned two people who the Lord took. One was Enoch, and the other was Elijah. God took them, but He took them alive, not dead! The exact phrase to use when a believer dies is that " He went home to be with the Lord" . He went! Many believers are going home to meet the Lord in an untimely death; it is not that the Lord took them!

> " *For then must he often have suffered since the foundation of the world: but now once in the end of the world hath he appeared to put away sins, by the sacrifice of himself.*
>
> *And as it is appointed unto men once to die, but after this the judgement:"*
>
> *So Christ was once offered to bear the sins of many; and unto them that look for him shall he appear the second time without sin unto salvation"*
>
> *Hebrews 9:26-28*

Many believers quote " it is appointed unto men once to die..." thinking that God has appointed the day, time and year every individual upon the face of the earth will die. That it does not matter what we do, when that fixed day, time and year comes, off we go. Well, that is wrong! A big X to that.

First of all we need to understand the key word here. That word is once. The Bible is talking here about dying one time and not about a time to die.

You might then say, preacher, well Ecclesiastes says that there is " a time to die" . Well let's examine that scripture and see what it is saying:

" To every thing there is a season, and a time to every purpose under the heaven:

A time to be born and a time to die, a time to plant, and a time to pluck up that which is planted".

Ecclesiastes 3:1-2

This scripture is talking about times and seasons. Just as there is a right time to be born, which is precisely after nine months of conception, similarly so, there is a right time or season to die. A child coming out before its time is a premature baby. It is not born in its right time, similarly so can a man die prematurely. It is just the same with harvest. A corn of grain needs to be harvested full-grown.

This scripture is not suggesting that God has set a time say for Mr. John to die on Sunday 2 July 1998 at exactly 4:00 PM. Absolutely not! What He is saying is that there is a right season to die. What we need to ask ourselves is, what season is it for a man to die? That is what I am going to tell you in this chapter.

" According to my earnest expectation and my hope, that in nothing I shall be ashamed, but that with all boldness, as always, so now also Christ shall be magnified in my body, whether it be by life, or by death.

For to me to live is Christ, and to die is gain.

But if I live in the flesh, this is the fruit of my labour: yet what I shall choose I wot not.

For I am in a strait betwixt two, having a desire to depart, and to be with Christ, which is far better:

Nevertheless to abide in the flesh is more needful for you.

And having this confidence, I know that I shall abide and continue with you all for the furtherance and joy of faith;"

Philippians 1:20-25

From this portion of scriptures, we see that Paul had a say as to whether he live of die. At first he did not know what to do, whether he should die and go to be with the Lord, (which is far better) or be with the saints and continue with them (for the furtherance and joy of faith).

We see him then deciding to live and not die because the philippian Church needs him. We then see him choosing to live. The choice was his. Though at first he was undecided about it, eventually he chose to stay. Brethren, you can choose to die young and leave the rest of the work to us to do and go to be with the Lord or you can stay for the furtherance and joy of faith.

Whenever you choose to live or die let Christ be magnified in it. There is a right season to die and there is a wrong season to die. There is a right way to die and there is a wrong way to die. Do not die with sickness and disease; do not die as a fool or an evildoer. Let your death glorify God.

You might ask about those saints who were killed for the gospel. What would you say about their death preacher? Well, lets see what the word had to say about them:

" Who through faith subdued, kingdoms, wrought righteousness, obtained promises, stopped the mouth of lions,

Quenched the violence of the fire, escaped the edge of the sword, out of weakness were made strong, waxed valiant in fight, turned to flight the armies of the aliens.

Women received their dead back to life again: and others were tortured, not accepting deliverance; that they might obtain a better resurrection:"

Hebrews 11:33-35

Two kinds of people we should be talking about here. The one, through faith overcame death threatening circumstances and even death itself: (women received their dead back to life again).

We also need to consider those who died or were killed. Some of them would have died very young. The last verse told us that these people " refused deliverance". They could have chosen to refuse death like the others, but they choose not to. Their reason was that they might obtain a better resurrection. From scriptures, we know that there is a martyr's crown and they want to obtain that.

> " *Fear none of those things which thou shalt suffer: behold, the devil will cast some of you into prison, that they may be tried; and ye shall have tribulation ten days: be thou faithful unto death, and I will give you a crown of life"*
> *Rev 2:10*

We must also know that these people glorified God in their death, the choice is still ours. They refused deliverance. We can choose to die a martyr's death or we can choose to live for Christ. At one time in Paul's life he choose to stay and at the last he chooses to go. Our duty is not to judge other Christian's death. If a Christian is tired of this sinful world and wants to go and be with the Lord, it is his choice. He has not sinned, but the choice to live is also yours:

" I call heaven and earth to record this day against you, that I have set before you life and death, blessing and cursing: therefore choose life, that both you and your seed may live:"

Deuteronomy 30:19

A Right Season To Die

I believe that the right season to die is a good old age. This is a period of time after you have lived your life in full. That is the time to die. You must see your children's children at least two generations before you die. This is your portion from the Lord if you would believe it.

" Thou shalt come to thy grave in a full age, like as a shock of corn cometh in its season.

Lo this, we have searched it, so it is; hear it, and know thou it for thy good" .

Job 5:26-27

" To every thing there is a season, and a time to every purpose under the heaven:

A time to born and a time to die; a time to plant, and a time to pluck up that which was planted".

Ecclesiastes 3:1-2

A Wrong Time to Die

There is also a wrong time to die. People do die a premature death. They do die before their time, the scriptures teach that.

> " *Be not over much wicked, neither be thou foolish: why shouldest thou die before thy time?*

Ecclesiastes 7:17

> " *...Bloody and deceitful men shall not live half their days; but I trust in thee*

Psalm 55:23b

By the mouth of two or three witnesses of scriptures, it has been established that some people die before their time and others live half their days. The wicked die before their time as well as the foolish.

Conditions For Longevity of Life

Let's look at God's prescribed way of living long upon this earth. These are not my ideas, but God's. These are the Biblical keys for longevity of life. We need to understand these things if we are to live our lives to the full on this earth.

Know that it is God's will for you to live long in this earth. The Devil would have you to be ignorant concerning this, and God's children are indeed destroyed for lack of knowledge. You can't act upon what you do not know aout, so, know that longevity of life belongs to you.

Stay on the word of God

You need to be obedient to the word of God at all times. Go according to the principles of the kingdom of God. Do not turn away from them. Be also obedient to the inner voice and witness of the Holy Spirit within you because longevity of life also depends on your obedience to the Holy Spirit within you. Listen to the voice of the Spirit when you drive, eat, play, etc. Disobedience to that voice can cost you your life.

Prov.3: 1-2, Prov. 9:10-11, Job 12:12; prov.14; 9:11; 10:27

Passive Christians will not make longevity of life, only active Christians will. Those who hide under the philosophy that " whatever happens to their lives is God's will for them without you having nothing to do about it" , will not make it for this blessing of God. Longevity of life is for those who will say Lord, this is your will, there is a price to pay, and I will pay it.

"Wherefore be not unwise, but understanding what the will of the Lord is" .

Ephesians 5:17

" And ye shall serve the LORD your God, and he shall bless thy bread, and thy water; and I will take sickness away from the midst of thee.

There shall nothing cast their young, nor be barren, in thy land: the number of thy days I will fulfil"

Exodus 23:25-26

If we serve the Lord, these are the blessings we receive from God:

- He will bless our bread and our water (free them from poison)
- He will take sickness away from our midst (divine health)
- The number of our days He will fulfil (Longevity of life)
- No miscarriages or premature babies (no premature death)

The food we eat and drink, and human interferences with nature are the main causes of sickness and death in our communities. If we serve our God, He will keep us from all of these.

You must learn to honour Authority

You must practise honouring and respecting those who are older and in authority over you, this of course is inclusive of your parents. This is the first commandment with a promise.

Exodus 20:12; Ephesians 6:2-3; Proverbs. 10:27

Watch your tongue

Speak good things and you will receive good things. Your tongue can get you into trouble that can cost you your life. Do not be a busybody in other men's matter, and do not be a talebearer. Strife can also get you into trouble. Longevity of life is not entirely up to God; you've also got a part to play in it. You are also responsible for the length of life you'll live. Though God is sovereign man also has a responsibility. God's sovereignty and man's responsibility brings the promise of God into effect.

Psalm 34:12-13; 1Pet 3:10

Know how to walk in peace and rest

Do not get depressed or wallow in self-piety. Kick depression out of your life. Depression is a killer; it encourages self-pity and suicidal tendencies. Also keep away from anger, hatred and strife. They cause distress and distress is not good for your health. Learn to deal with pressure and stress. They do shorten life span. Guard your life from them.

It is also good that you take your rest in sleep and quietness. Leave work for a while, go somewhere and just relax. By relax I mean no reading, no exercise, nothing whatsoever. Just lie down and sleep. Relax your mind and just wait on God. Just lay back and let God speak to you.

1Pet 5:7, Matthew 6:25,31,34; Psalm 55:22

Eat well and eat blessed food

We are told in God's word that He will bless our mouth with good things, so that our youth will be renewed like that of an eagle (paraphrased). We are also promised that God would bless our drink and food as we eat them. What we eat also has a great deal to do with a good health though good health is not entirely up to eating good things.

We need to believe God for good food so that our health would be renewed day by day. Rest and bodily exercises are also vital for our health. Watch the things you eat. Too much fat is not good for your health. Do some fasting it makes health spring forth speedily.

We also need to ask the Lord to bless our food and drink. Many of our food out there contain a lot of things that can kill us. Make it a practise to bless your food all the time before you eat. If you eat blessed food, you are guaranteed of the necessary nutrients for a good long life.

1Timothy 4:8; Isaiah 58:8

Be a fighter

There are many things out there that can try our faith, but you must be a fighter. Do not give up on sickness and disease; fight it because God has promised not only to heal you, but to keep sickness and disease away from you.

You might have made a mistake in life and you are now suffering for it. If you had confessed your sin to God, you can be well assured of His forgiveness. Forgive yourself now and get out of that sickness you are in and finish the work the Lord gave you to do.

Do not be idle. Do the work God has given you to do. Be a visionary. Always have something to live for. Occupy till He comes back to reward you for your faithfulness. The labourers are few; keep on keeping on, and fight until you reach that good old age.

Death is an Enemy

Death is not a blessing rather it is a curse. It is not of God, it is an enemy. The Bible says that it will be the last enemy that would be destroyed. Some people are said to be healed in death. Death never heals anyone.

" The last enemy that shall be destroyed is death"

1Corinthians 15:26

" And death and hell are cast into the lake of fire. This is the second death"

Revelation 20:14

" And the Lord shall wipe away all tears from their eyes; and there shall be no more death, neither sorrow, nor crying, neither shall their be anymore pain: for the former thing are passed away"

Revelation 21:4

How long is Long?

I believe the question that one need to answer is how long is long and how old is old? Some people think that after they have passed 40 years they are now on the down side of life. Others think that at 18, they are old enough. Now lets see if God has prescribed an approximate maximum that we can believe Him for. I believe that approximate maximum is prescribed in the word of God, and that maximum is 120 years.

" And the LORD said, my spirit shall not always strive

with man, for that he also is flesh: yet his days shall be an hundred and twenty years"

Genesis 6:4

Before the flood people lived until nine hundred and sixty nine years. When wickedness began to fill the earth, (can you imagine people living eight to nine centuries doing wickedness), God had to shorten the life span of mankind. He then gave us a maximum of 120 years. God has never changed that anywhere in scripture that I know of.

After the flood, man's years start to decrease from Shem being 600 years old, to 120 years when Moses died. Others even died younger than that. Some believer would think the maximum is seventy years. This is not so. Let's examine that Psalm of Moses and see what he was talking about when he mentioned seventy years.

" The days of our years are three score and ten; and if by reason of strength they be fourscore years, yet is their strength labour and sorrow; for it is soon cut off, and we fly away" .

Psalm 90:10

Moses was in remorse here. He was in mourning

here. He was talking about a people consumed under anger and wrath as a result of their sins. *Numbers 14:22-34* explains who those people were. Moses was lamenting about the Children of Israel dying in the wilderness as a result of their unbelief, when they brought an evil report of the land to the people.

God told them that that generation would all die in the wilderness and it is only those who were twenty and under who will enter the promise land. God said that they would all die and their children will wander for forty years in the wilderness.

If we add forty years to the years of those who were over twenty that should die in the wilderness, they would be between seventy and eighty years before they will soon die. God was in no way saying that the maximum years of all mankind should be seventy. No not at all. So to be old is not forty, that's only one third of your life, believe God for a maximum, 120 years.

In fact, God said that He would satisfy us with long life, so live until you are satisfied. If you are not yet satisfied with the life you have lived, ask God to add more to your years.

"With long life will I satisfy him and show him my salvation"

Psalm 91:16

IMPORTANT

Jesus does not want only to heal your body; He also wants to save your spirit too. He wants to give you a new life. He wants your heart saved as well as your body saved. He wants, after you have lived a good long life, to have you with Him in Heaven when you die. Do you want to accept Him as your Saviour and Lord? You can say this prayer with me:

The Sinner's Prayer

Dear God in Heaven, have mercy on me a sinner. I repent of my sins. With my heart I believe Jesus died for my sins according to the Scriptures. With my mouth I confess that Jesus is my Lord and personal Saviour.

I open my heart to you Jesus. Come into my life and make me a new person. I believe you have come into my life and I believe you are my Lord and Saviour. Thank you Lord for giving me eternal life in Jesus' name. Amen

Congratulations

Congratulations! Welcome into the family of God! Your name is written in Heaven. Sin shall not have dominion over you. You are now a ruler over sin, sickness and the devil. Now start reading the word of God and grow in your new life.

Live a life of prayer and tell someone about the saving and healing power of God. Find a Church that believes the word as you have been taught, and serve Him there. God bless you.

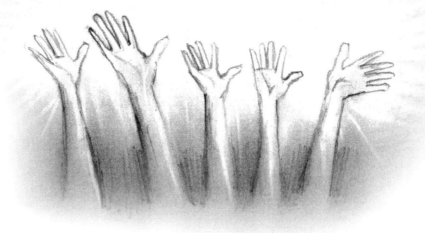

Testimonies

I have tried to catalogue 7 testimonies of healing in my ministry for the purpose of this book. God has healed countless people in over 15 years of my ministry in Sierra Leone, Italy and The United Kingdom. Here are 7 of such healings written down by the people who experienced them.

Abnormal Cells in the mouth of womb disappear.

Praise the Lord Almighty who is the God who heals all diseases. Had it not been the Lord of Hosts that delivered me, I would have been battling with cancer but I thank God Almighty who has set His word above His name. When God says, " you are healed", so be it.

I did a smear test, which is a normal procedure in the United Kingdom, and the result showed that I had abnormal cells in the mouth of my womb. The doctor said that if I fail to have it treated, it would lead to cervical cancer.

I told my pastor and we prayed for God to heal me. We later thanked God for His healing power. I believed that God had performed a surgery in my womb, however; we needed the doctor to confirm it. The doctor booked me to do a Coloposcy on the 16th of August 2000. God proved to the doctors that He is a miracle working God. The doctor did the examination again and could not find any trace of abnormal cell in my womb even with the microscope he had that could detect the minutest cell in my body.

The doctor and his nurse were very puzzled. The first test showed abnormal cells present in my womb but now, they could find nothing in my womb or the mouth of my womb. The doctor then took a sample from my womb to do a lab test on it. He had little knowledge that when the Lord performs a miracle it is done to perfection. Later on they wrote me a letter to say that I need no further treatment. Praise God!

I cannot thank the Lord enough for His healing power and for His greatness. He is the Lord Almighty and He performs miracles to perfection. Praise the Lord. Amen.

This healing was done on one of my members in my Church in London in August 2000. The Sister declined to include her name in the testimony but if you for any reason want to verify the healing you can contact us and we can contact her. She will be more than willing to share her testimony with you with supporting evidences. All we can say concerning her is that she is an accountant and a degree holder.

We thank God for healing her and we give all the glory to God. May all who read this with similar problems receive faith to be healed?

May our God who healed this sister heal you of your plague, in Jesus' name, Amen.

With this healing, we know that the prayer of faith shall save the sick according to the book of James chapter 5:15

Healed of an irregular Menstrual Cycle

I am in my thirties and I stopped having my monthly menstrual cycle for the past three (3) years. I was very worried about this and for this cause went to the hospital many times. The doctors gave me a lot of different kinds of medication, which never did the job.

I started going to Church and praying that God would heal me since medical science could not help me. My Pastor declared a twenty-one (21) days praying and fasting for breakthrough for the entire Church which I took part in. At first I was very hesitant to go through the fasting but God spoke to me and said if I go through it, He will heal me, so I finally gave in to it.

On the second week of the prayer and fasting for my healing the fasting became very difficult for me. I denied the Devil of the victory as I persisted in prayer. As it was getting late that evening, my stomach began to hurt me very badly that I couldn't go to work that evening. I decided to take a shower thinking that this will help relieve me of the pain. As soon as I enter the bathtub something just drop from the inside of me into the tub with a thumbing sound.

It looks like a very big clot of blood. Immediately, the pain was gone and I started seeing my menstrual period again. Ever since, my menstrual cycle is normal and I give praise and glory to God for His healing power. Thank you Jesus for the wonderful healing you gave me. Amen

This is another account of healing that took place in my Church in England, which I pioneered, and Pastor for eight (8) years. This sister is one of the ushers in the Church and also Sunday school teacher. Her name is Laurine Cole and she is also a Chef for one of the offices in the West end of London.

Jesus taught us that there are some kinds of deliverances, which come about, only by prayer and fasting. This is a vivid example of such kind. You are encouraged to pray and fast for healing and God will hasten to perform His word for your life. Matthew 17:21

Minister healed of Atopic Eczema

In 1954, at the age of 6 months I developed eczema. In those days there was no proper treatment. Some of my earliest memories are of my mother trying out ointments and creams on me, some of which hurt badly. I had to be bandaged because I bled a lot, and the bandages stuck to me. Often my pyjamas stuck to my skin and I had to be sat in the bath with my clothes on to soften the scabs. I used to scratch so badly at night that one doctor suggested I should be tied hand and foot to the bed at night. It drove me so mad with frustration that I would fight myself free.

When I was 5 or 6 I remember my father carrying me through the streets of London (my skin was too stiff with crusts to move), to visit a Harley Street specialist. As a result of this I began to get some proper treatment at the Great Ormond Street Children's Hospital but there was no cure for atopic eczema.

At school I was always different, because I was the only child who had to leave the class to get bandaged. Getting undressed for sport or swimming was excruciating. I felt ashamed. As I got older I was bullied, and some children said really cruel things. I tried to ignore it.

After all, it was the only skin I'd ever known. Even so, I would some-times burst out with a " Why me?" in the vague direction of God.

I became a Christian at 18, and four years later I joined the church I still belong to. Ointments and baths were keeping my skin under some kind of control, but if the skin got infected, it flared up out of control. In 1983 I was hospitalised three times. On countless occasions I received prayer, but with no effect. At times I really believed it would happen, but nothing ever changed. It got to the stage where I no longer believed any-thing would happen. I felt I was living a lie. My disease was broadcast-ing to everyone around that God couldn't heal today.

In May 1999 a sister in my church gave herself to pray specifically for my situation. She felt God say to her that the root was demonic and that I should get prayer from Desmond Thomas of Flaming Evangelical Ministries, who is a good friend of mine. So I made an appointment and in early June I went to see him and his wife Mary in London.

When they prayed and named a spirit of infirmity, I felt a pain and nausea in my stomach. I was fully conscious, worshipping the Lord. In fact, I was able to tell Desmond what was happening. I was lying on the floor shaking and groaning, and I clearly sensed something evil moving up my body as far as my throat, and then leaving me. I felt a deep peace from God.

For the next fortnight the symptoms seemed as bad as ever, but I knew absolutely that the power behind it had been removed. So I kept declaring this aloud. I stopped using the steroid creams I had been on for 40 years, and just used my emulsifiers. Gradually the texture changed, the itch subsided and the redness disappeared. I am now com-pletely clear from the neck downwards and have been for over a year.

Only my scalp continues to need treatment, but I know that Jesus healed me totally, and soon I will have a normal skin all over. All praise to our mighty Saviour and Lord, Jesus Christ!

Trevor Saxby, Senior Leader, Jesus Fellowship Church, Milton Keynes.

This is a vivid example of a sickness caused by demonic spirits, Praise God for His healing!

Womb Extraction Operation Cancelled

A lady called me from United States of America in early 2000 and was very worried because doctors have diagnosed cyst and fibroid in her womb which they said would not allow her to become pregnant. In fact she was told that they would have to remove her womb altogether.

She was very troubled because her hope of having a baby was only a dream now. When she called me on the phone (someone gave her my number) she was very troubled and asked if I could pray for her. I took the time to share with her some of the things I have written in this book. Her faith grew and she believed that she would be healed. We agreed and prayed for her healing.

The day she phoned me was the day prior to her operation. The next day she called me and said that when they opened her up they could not find neither cyst not fibroid in her womb and that her womb was in perfect order. Praise the Lord! The prayer of faith would save the sick and if any two of us shall agree as touching anything we shall ask of our Father in Heaven, it shall be done. Amen

Barrenness Gone

A midwife came to our Church one day very desperate of having a baby. Her husband is a Gynaecologist. When she came to us to pray for her, her husband laughed. He said to her, " Of all people you should know that you could not have a baby". We have done all the tests and every other thing we can do for you to have a baby but you could not. She also had fibroid problems.

Through talking to her I observed she had a demonic problem. Through my interview of her I diagnosed that there is a strong demonic spirit preventing her from having a baby. There was an invincible presence around her especially when she is alone and in the night in her dream he would always appear to her attack and abuse her.

She was not saved so I challenged her to receive Jesus as her saviour and Lord, which she did. I invited her to come for deliverance ministration, which she did. Whilst praying for her she fell and felt something left her body. Instantly she was delivered.

To cut a long story short, she now has two healthy children. God is so good and He is good all the time. He is faithful to His word and He still confirms his word with signs and wonders following. Amen.

Deaf and dumb healed

These two miracles took place early in my healing ministry. They have always astounded me. We had rented a small Church in the town where we started our first Church. We invited people to come to the meetings, which we announced to be a healing and deliverance crusade.

We spent a lot of time praying and fasting for the meeting and the Church hall was packed full with people. Miracles started to happen. A set of twins was brought to me to be prayed for. One of them was dumb and the other deaf. The power of the Lord was present to heal. After praying for them I started to talk to the deaf one and asked him to repeat what I said.

Praise the Lord; he started to repeat my words back to me, hallelujah! He was healed. The lady who brought them told me that he has never done that before. Praise the Lord for that miracle.

The other twin brother then began to speak back to me as I asked him to do so. That day was one of the most awesome days in my life. I thank God for using my in that miracle. It then gave me more faith and confidence in God to do exceedingly abundantly above all that I could ask or imagined.

Twins from a cemented Womb

A childhood friend of my wife came to our Church. In search of a child she asked us to pray for her. She was having difficulties in child bearing. She will see her period sometimes only ones a year. Her first boyfriend left her because she couldn't have a baby. Her enemies called her "cemented womb" thinking she wouldn't have a child.

She later had a miscarriage and a baby induced because he died in the womb only few months old. She lost all hope and faith in God and blamed God for all her troubles. In her grief she said one day that if Satan would give her a child she would serve him rather than serving God.

We never gave up on her neither did God gave up on her. We encouraged her to commit herself to the Lord and to her she need to live godly and righteously before God. She was living with a man and they were not married. She then got married. One day she came to the Church and the Spirit of God told me to call her up and pray for her. After finished praying for her, the Holy Ghost told me she is going to give birth to twins a boy and a girl. God told me He is going to give her double for all her troubles.

To cut a long story short, God did gave her twins (a boy and a girl), that's how a cemented womb gave birth to twins, Hallelujah, Amen!